This Is *Not* Your Mother's Menopause

VILLARD

NEW YORK

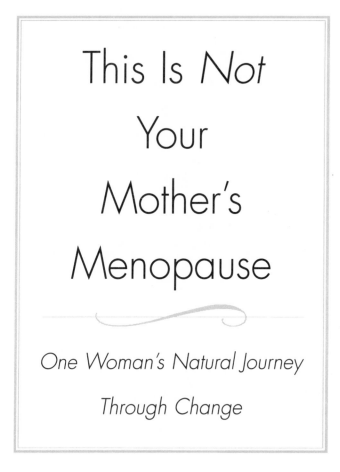

This Is *Not* Your Mother's Menopause

One Woman's Natural Journey

Through Change

TRISHA   POSNER

All rights reserved under International and Pan-American Copyright Conventions.
Published in the United States by Villard Books,
a division of Random House, Inc., New York, and
simultaneously in Canada by Random House
of Canada Limited, Toronto.

VILLARD BOOKS and colophon are registered trademarks of Random House, Inc.

Library of Congress Cataloging-in-Publication Data
Posner, Trisha.
This is not your mother's menopause: one woman's natural journey through change /
Trisha Posner.
p.   cm.
Includes bibliographical references.
ISBN 0-375-50398-6
1. Menopause—Popular works. I. Title.

RG186 .P665 2000
618.1'75 21; aa05 10-27—dc99   99-055033

Random House website address: www.atrandom.com

Printed in the United States of America on acid-free paper

2 4 6 8 9 7 5 3

First Edition

Book design by JAM DESIGN

To my soul mate, Gerald,
the only person who really knows me

This Is Not *Your Mother's Menopause* is the personal story of how I dealt with the choices that confronted me when I unexpectedly learned I was in menopause. It follows my search to discover whether there was an alternative beyond the American Medical Association's sanctioned regimen of hormone replacement therapy and doing nothing while my body slowly deteriorated. Although my gynecologist was adamant that hormone replacement was the only reasonable choice, I was not so easily convinced. Since my mother, and two aunts, had had breast cancer, it was a risk I refused to ignore. While I knew there were no proven means of reducing breast cancer risk, I did not want to do anything that worsened my odds.

Despite my gynecologist's advice, I was determined that, if there were another option, I would find it. From plowing through books and articles at the New York Public Library's reading room to searching Internet medical discussion sites, I slowly pieced together a broad list of natural remedies that promised either to alleviate some of my symptoms or to stop deterioration of bones, loss of skin elasticity, reduction of libido, memory loss, and the rest of the catastrophes that are supposed to happen if you don't take hormones.

I certainly don't object to the choice made by millions of women to use hormone replacement to deal with the changes wrought by menopause. For many it is a viable way of handling this passage. Some implicitly trust their doctors' recommendations that estrogen is a wonder drug. And obviously for many it does work. But I believe that too many women think hormone replacement is their *only* salvation, and if they do not take it then their sole choice is to do nothing and wait for the "ravages" of menopause to begin. I now know there are alternatives, and I am proof of that. When I started my research, I was soon convinced that this midlife passage had served as a real wake-up call not only to concentrate on my health but also to prepare myself emotionally for the second half of my life. During my journey I did discover natural remedies that alleviated my discomforting symptoms while preventing heart disease and osteoporosis. There are exercise and beauty regimens that not only helped combat the possible loss of muscle tissue, drying skin, and thinning hair, but actually helped me get into the best shape of my life.

I do not know if my program will work for others, but it did work for me. And my journey of self-discovery and defiance in the face of my doctor's strident advice shows that, as women, we do have choices other than the narrow ones commonly presented. Making uninformed decisions regarding our bodies may be more dangerous than doing nothing at all. And since news in menopause and women's health changes rapidly—and conflicting medical studies create confusion—being an informed consumer is critical.

In *The Silent Passage,* Gail Sheehy's groundbreaking book on menopause, she highlighted the depressing record of most physicians when it comes to this phase of a woman's life. Many doctors are simply not up-to-date on the various and often subtle biological changes women undergo during menopause. Dismissing most of our symptoms as inconsequential, or as merely psychological, doctors usually reach for a simple cure-all. However, each of us has different risk factors based on our family histories and lifestyles, and each will experience varying problems with the onset of menopause. Some women have a particularly difficult passage, while a few sail through almost symptom free. The very notion that a single treatment could work in all these diverse cases seems silly on its face, but it is precisely what the medical establishment wants us to believe. Instead of critically analyzing each woman's individual needs, lifestyle, and risks, too many doctors have the knee-jerk response of merely prescribing hormones.

More than 20 million baby boomers will enter menopause during the next ten years. As modern women, we take control of our lives in a myriad of ways that our mothers never contemplated. Approaching menopause, the one journey in life that we all share, should be no different. Our mothers were largely silent about what happened to them as they passed through this midlife change. But a new generation of women has already started to break the wall of silence. More information and more alternatives are available than ever before. We have the ability to control naturally every aspect of this inevitable woman's passage. There is tremendous strength and satisfaction in assuming more responsibility for our own well-being and emerging from menopause healthier and more vigorous than ever.

This book is for informational purposes only. It revolves around a program of exercise, diet, and nutritional supplements that worked for me, but since I am not a doctor, I don't know if it would work for anyone else. I don't think any woman should embark on a new regimen without first checking with her own physician.

Also, I want to make it clear that I don't have any commercial interest in any product, treatment, or organization mentioned in this book. Whatever I've used in helping myself master menopause was a result of trial and error and, finally, settling on whatever worked best.

ACKNOWLEDGMENTS

The idea for this book came to me after I watched, and simmered, through a five-part television series about menopause in which there was no discussion about any alternatives to estrogen replacement therapy. Well into my own holistic regimen by then, I sat down and knocked out an angry proposal to my husband Gerald's editor at Random House, Bob Loomis. Bob is more than an editor; he has become a trusted friend and adviser to us over the years. It was his encouragement and counsel that helped me refine my early scattered ideas for a book.

As the proposal made the rounds at Random House, I was fortunate that it landed on the desk of Bruce Tracy, the editorial director of Villard. Bruce immediately understood why this personal journal was so different from the dozens of other books about menopause. I could not have asked for a better editor. Although I had worked closely with Gerald on seven books, this was my first solo project, and it did take some time before I was really comfortable. Bruce— blessed with great intelligence and a wonderful sense of humor—guided me patiently, always showing considerable enthusiasm and commitment. I owe him a big thank-you.

Publishing at Random House/Villard was perfect for me, as I knew many of the people there from Gerald's work. It was like coming home to see a group of dear and trusted friends. Art director Daniel Rembert made the creative work on the book jacket seem so simple—and he eased my apprehension about having my picture on the cover. I am grateful to him for his good wit and fine artistic eye. Assistant editor Oona Schmid was always extremely helpful with my many and varied requests, and her professionalism never flagged, even when tested. Deborah Aiges, vice president and creative director, took time from her busy duties to read my manuscript. Not only did she have suggestions that made the book better, but I greatly appreciated her early zeal. I thank her for her honesty and support. Susan Brown, the copy editor, had a keen eye for tightening my prose while maintaining the integrity of my voice. Beth Pearson, who has overseen the editorial production on three of Gerald's books, is a friend. I knew hard work and probing questions were her trademark, but still I could not have foreseen how helpful she was in polishing the manuscript.

As I worked on this book, I realized that much of my success in tackling menopause was due to my fierce determination to refuse to be told by my doctor that I could not do it on my own. That rebellious spirit and my strength of will are definitely gifts from my fabulous mother, Sadie.

And my aunt Rose taught me as a child to fight for whatever I wanted. This book is bittersweet for me, since I am ecstatic that my mother—a vibrant breast cancer survivor—is here to enjoy my first publication, but I am deeply disappointed that Aunt Rose passed away unexpectedly at the age of eighty-nine, just as I was putting the final touches to my manuscript. She would have relished this book.

And finally, to my darling love, Gerald. We are blessed to have a very special bond, one that is completely satisfying and nurturing. I cannot imagine being without him, and I know I could not have done this book on my own. Gerald has infused me with the belief that I could do anything I put my mind to, and he literally worked as my partner from the first draft through the final proofreading. It sounds hackneyed to say there would be no book without him, but in this case it is true. His belief in me is something I never take for granted. I am so delighted he is my eternal partner.

CONTENTS

This Is *Not*
Your
Mother's
Menopause

"I'm What?!"

"YOUR mother has breast cancer." Months of her complaints of terrible stomachaches and a general malaise had led me to speculate about many ailments that might afflict my eighty-four-year-old mother, but somehow breast cancer was never on the list. I had trouble concentrating on what else the doctor—six thousand miles away in Britain—was saying, my mind already racing about possible treatments and fretting over how scared my mother must be. Although the doctor kept talking, her words seemed to run together and I let the telephone slip away from my ear. I stared out the window of my San Francisco hotel room. A thick blanket of fog saturated the city and our twentieth-floor room seemed as if it were suspended in clouds. It added to the already surreal effect of getting this disturbing news, only a few years after my mother's sister—an aunt who had helped raise me—had been diagnosed with the same cancer.

"What's the matter?" my husband, Gerald, whispered. He put down his newspaper and walked over when he sensed that something was terribly amiss.

"Mum has breast cancer."

"What!"

He had been wonderfully supportive through my mother's recent illnesses and had helped prepare me for possible bad news, but not for this. When I finally got off the phone with the doctor, and before I called my mother, my husband gently kissed me. "She's a survivor," he said. "If anyone can pull through this, she will." I nodded, wanting to believe that his confidence was not misplaced.

"And if there is any silver lining," he continued, "aren't you glad you made the choice you did last spring?"

For a moment I had almost forgotten. Over a year ago I'd had my annual physical in my doctor's office on the Upper East Side of Manhattan. Everything had seemed fine. Cholesterol was low, blood pressure normal, and vital signs good. A week later he telephoned.

"Your blood test just came back."

His voice seemed tense, but I thought I might be imagining it since a call from my doctor was unexpected.

"Anything wrong?"

"No, no. But I did want you to know that your FSH [follicle-stimulating hormone] serum levels came back at one hundred ten, and the normal range is between two and ten."

"What does that mean?"

"It means you are in full-blown menopause."

Different, and obviously much less frightening than hearing about my mother's cancer, but just as startling. I was forty-six. I had read articles and seen documentaries about perimenopause—the several-year span of wildly varying hormonal levels that precedes full menopause—and had always expected that I would get some distinct warnings. There were none I could immediately think of. And somehow I felt I was a little too young. My mother had passed through a moderately difficult change of life in her mid-fifties. Two maternal aunts were also in their fifties when they were in menopause. Maybe, believing it might be a decade away, I had merely put off any serious thought of it, conveniently not paying attention to any signs.

"Are you sure?" I asked my doctor.

"No doubt about it, Trisha," he said, trying to be reassuring but only adding a little to my angst. "Your numbers are so high, you are well into the change. It's time to make a quick appointment with your gynecologist."

The only real concern I had about menopause was that it brought to a head my long-standing indecision regarding hormone replacement therapy. No longer was estrogen simply the subject of a heated luncheon debate with a group of girlfriends, none of us menopausal but all with strong opinions pro and con. Now I faced an imminent decision: Was estrogen right for me, or could I pass through menopause without it?

My gynecologist of nearly twenty years left no doubt about the choice I should make if I was—in his words—"an intelligent, well-informed woman who wanted to ensure that her health remained good and that she was vital for her later years." That was his not very subtle way of recommending an immediate program of estrogen and progesterone. If I did not start promptly, he warned, a host of virtually cataclysmic events would overtake my body.

"You are in complete uterine failure," he said grimly, as though he were informing me about some fatal condition. "This isn't good at all. Your blood test reveals that your estrogen is gone. Your bones are probably already losing mass. You have to worry about osteoporosis." He had zeroed in on one of my major apprehensions; since I'm allergic to almost all dairy products, I've always resorted to supplements for my calcium.

He did not, however, let me think about that for very long before adding new concerns. "Your heart is no longer getting any protective effects from your hormones," he announced. "Your memory will worsen. Your metabolism is going to get sluggish, and fat is going to start depositing as you lose muscle tissue. You have to start a program now."

"But my aunt has breast cancer, and it concerns me," I protested weakly.

He waved his arm in a large dismissive arc. "Rubbish. More women die of heart disease than ever die of breast cancer. The studies that raise fear about estrogen are biased and wrong. Estrogen doesn't increase your risk of breast cancer. If you let your fear stop you, you will be sorry for the toll your body will suffer. You really don't have another choice. Doing nothing is negligent."

Despite, or maybe because of, his persistence, I decided that day to be obstinate, and refused to immediately start a program of long-term hormone replacement, even if the odds of increased breast and uterine cancer were small. I was not willing to play Russian roulette with my health, no matter how small the risk, at least not until I had satisfied myself there was no other alternative. Moreover, my mother and her sisters had passed through menopause without hormone replacement, and they lived on their own, healthy and mentally vibrant well into their eighties. I mentioned this to my doctor.

"It's a mistake, Trisha," he said. "The benefits of estrogen are too important to ignore. Every month you wait sets you further back."

"I'll be back in a few months," I told him. "Let's see what develops."

From Studio 54 to Menopause

WHEN I left my gynecologist's office that warm summer day, I was convinced only that I had bought myself some extra time and probably just delayed the inevitable decision to say yes to his hormone replacement program. Although I usually have no problem making quick decisions, even on important issues, somehow I wanted to procrastinate over whether I would become estrogen dependent.

As I walked home, I passed a record store in midtown. Gloria Gaynor's disco classic "I Will Survive" was blasting at megadecibels through the open doors. I stopped for a moment and caught my reflection in the large plate-glass window. A sheet of blue cellophane covered the window, and the way the sun bounced off the glass, it distorted my image, almost as if I were standing in front of a trick mirror in a fun house. The slightly squashed features and bloated face matched my mood. For a few moments on that busy New York street, I must have seemed a strange sight, just standing in front of the store, seemingly staring at the array of electronic goodies, although my focus was really just on my own reflection.

I don't know if other women who are suddenly told they are in menopause experience anything similar, but I was swept by this rather nostalgic wave as I stood there. The mind is a marvel that can conjure up some pretty strange diversions when you don't want to think directly about a pressing problem. And at that moment I did not want to think about the choice my gynecologist had given me. Instead, the song entranced me, and although it was very upbeat, it made me feel sad.

I had moved to New York from London in the spring of 1978. At the time I was designing a men's clothing line, and as a twenty-seven-year-old, single British girl, I fell into a hip, mostly gay, New York fashion crowd. I soon moved into an apartment in a new West Fifty-seventh Street high-rise with one of my gay friends, Bill, an actor and model. Down the hallway, our neighbor was Marc Benecke, who turned out to be a doorman. That didn't sound very glamorous, until we discovered the door he ran was at the city's hottest nightclub, Studio 54. Every day I worked hard at my business, and several nights a week I was at Studio, dancing for hours. On weekends it was on to Fire Island, where Calvin Klein then held court, and there was more dancing in the Pines.

I had danced back then to Gloria Gaynor's song, and had also used it as a personal anthem during one particularly difficult breakup with a boyfriend. It brought back a lot of memories. Most of my dearest friends from that time, including my roommate Bill, had died of AIDS during the past two decades. You couldn't have been involved in fashion or the arts in New York since the late 1970s and not had the sad task of crossing out many cherished names from your address book. Bill, who had a wicked sense of humor and was obsessed with youthfulness, would have thought it quite hilarious that I was in menopause.

It seemed a hell of a long journey from those carefree nights at Studio, when my biggest decision was what to wear, to bearing the real responsibility of deciding whether I would put hormones into my body, possibly forever, or go my own route and try to find out if there were other answers. I moved my head a little to the right, and my face seemed even fatter in the window. Maybe that's how I'll look, I thought, if I don't start taking estrogen. If my gynecologist had this window in his office, he would easily scare all of us onto immediate hormone replacement.

When the music abruptly stopped, it was as if someone had pinched me out of a trance. I quickly walked down the block to one of my favorite coffee shops. A good dose of caffeine was sure to clear out the mental cobwebs and help wash away that bit of unusual nostalgia.

As I sat there sipping black coffee, I began thinking that possibly my test results were wrong. We had all heard stories where results were mistakenly swapped. Maybe what I needed instead of hormone replacement was another blood test. This diagnosis didn't sound right. The other night, while channel-surfing TV, I'd chanced upon a special on menopause. The hostess looked much more like Barbara Bush than like me. She seemed amiable enough, but the things she spoke about weren't directed to my generation, so I had quickly flipped to another channel. Yes, the more I thought about it, the more I was convinced I was right. Menopause? Not me.

"Are you busy or can you talk?" I yelled to Gerald as I walked into the apartment. He was typing away, working on a deadline for a magazine article. He more or less grunted, which I took to mean that he was busy. But I didn't want to wait to discuss this, so I marched into the library and stood next to him.

"Look at me," I commanded.

He stopped typing in mid-sentence and glanced up.

"Does this look like menopause?" I asked, holding my arms out and turning around so he could see my entire body. Before he could answer, I continued.

"You know, I've been thinking about it, and I think they're wrong about this menopause."

He gave me a look that suggested I was fishing for an unlikely explanation.

"Well, it's true," I continued. "Women just don't go into menopause without some symptoms. And I haven't had any."

"What about your headaches during the past six months?" he asked.

Yes, I had been suffering with bouts of often intense headaches, but I'd ascribed those to tension.

"A lot of people are headache sufferers. It doesn't mean much," I countered.

"Haven't you been asking me a lot recently, 'Is it hot in here, or is it me?' " he asked.

Occasionally I had felt warm, as though someone had turned up the heat, but I'd imagined only that my internal thermometer was somehow running off-kilter. And when I went to bed, I sometimes had to let my feet—which seemed to be burning up—stick out from under the blankets and sheets.

"Well . . ."

"And your breasts have been so tender," he continued, not giving me time for another excuse. Tenderness in my breasts was not something new, so I had paid little attention.

"What about your periods?" he asked. "You're the one who's been telling me that they haven't been on schedule for quite a while."

My periods had been irregular, heavy, and substantially shorter. I had even missed a couple. I had shrugged it off as the stress of modern living.

And he didn't mention it, but occasionally I had felt a little blue, something very unusual for me. After a recent trip to Memphis researching a book on the assassination of Martin Luther King, Jr., I had dubbed those few weeks "Memphis blues" because of a feeling of general malaise.

Suddenly, now that I focused on all the symptoms, I realized that my denial had been strong enough to smother any thought that I might be entering that inevitable midlife passage. Putting together this little list was somehow like figuring out a jigsaw puzzle that spelled out MENOPAUSE.

I plopped down in an overstuffed club chair. "Well, what the hell am I going to do?" I asked myself as much as Gerald.

I explained what my gynecologist had so strongly recommended. I didn't need to tell Gerald why I was hesitant about going so quickly on hormones, given my family history of breast cancer. It may be true that more women die of heart disease each year, but that didn't minimize the fact that nearly 200,000 American women are diagnosed annually with breast cancer, and almost 50,000 of us die from it each year. It is the most common women's cancer, and the longer we live the greater our chance of getting it is. For women in my age-group, thirty-five to fifty-four, it is the number-one cause of death. Even when it is caught early, and the prognosis is good, breast cancer often leaves physical and emotional scars that can take a long time to heal.

Gerald walked over, sat on the arm of my chair, and gently grabbed my shoulders. I felt very protected. "Nobody is better than you in researching every bit of information that exists on a subject," he said. "You've unearthed tons of news in archives and libraries around the world on everything from Nazi war criminals to assassins." It was true that, in working with Gerald on his books, I had enjoyed my role as a researcher, plowing through documents, interviews, and dusty files. I had always been interested in learning, so research wasn't really work for me, but something I relished.

"So, how is that going to help me now?"

"I think you need to approach this as a new project, but this time it's more important than anything you've done before, because this time it's about your health and our life together. You've got to research everything you can. That's the only way you're going to be satisfied that you're making the right decision about hormones. I don't know if they're right for you. Maybe they are. But I know you, and the only way you'll be comfortable is if you make sure on your own, and not just rely on a doctor's recommendation."

I knew he was right. I've always been someone who likes to control the events in her life. And as he was saying that, I realized that part of my problem with what my gynecologist had told me was that he presented menopause as a fait accompli, that my only choices were hormone replacement or slow and steady deterioration. Forcing me into a medical option that I was not sure was the best one was a sure way to make me rebel. At least if I did my research, and was satisfied he was right, I could deal with menopause as if I was in control.

"I'll help you," my husband said, his words breaking into my thoughts. "I'll help you this time around," he repeated, realizing that I had not been paying attention to him. "You're always there for me, helping me through every book. Now it's time for me to return the favor and help you figure out what's next." He leaned over and kissed me on the forehead.

I wasn't anxious anymore. I wasn't fighting the idea of whether or not I was in menopause. Now I was eager about something else: to log on to the Internet, to visit the library and my local bookstore, to start discovering what my options really were. It gave me a feeling of empowerment to know that I would review the information and decide what was best for my body. There would certainly be work ahead, but the payoff—making an informed decision at this critical midpoint of my life—would undoubtedly be worthwhile.

"It's a deal, partner," I said, smiling back at him. "Let's do it."

Studio 54 seemed very far away indeed.

THREE

The Secret in Our Closets

APPRECIATED my husband's support. It wasn't a surprise, since we had developed an extremely close bond during our sixteen years of marriage. We work together and spend virtually twenty-four hours a day with each other. Since he's my best friend, I expected no less. But I also knew that there was a real limit to what he could do for me. While he could be supportive during this transition, the physical changes were taking place in *my* body, and in the end I would have to be the one who made the adjustments. If there was a way to deal with possible deterioration from menopause without taking estrogen, I would have to be my own guinea pig, trying out various remedies to discover which, if any, worked.

The next day, while taking the subway to the main library, I looked around at the women in the packed car. It was a diverse group. There were several Asian schoolgirls giggling in one corner; a couple of middle-aged black women who seemed to be office workers were having an animated discussion; several older white women who were very casually dressed sat staring blankly ahead; and an Arabic girl, with her head covered by a traditional Muslim headdress, was reading a small book. But it was not the wonderful cultural diversity in that subway car that caught my attention that morning, but rather the realization that we, as women, are certain to have only one thing in common: menopause. Not even childbirth can compete, because some women never have children. But all of us—no matter our race, religion, or social standing—will, if we live long enough, be confronted with that inevitable midlife passage. And how many of us become passive, allowing menopause symptoms to run rampant because we have been told we have no other option, unless we control the process through hormones?

At the main library, after spending several hours in the stacks and card catalogues, I made what I thought was a good start at immersing myself in some of the nuances of menopause. Soon I was hidden behind a towering stack of periodicals, books, and rolls of microfilm. It did not take me long to realize that most of what I had initially pulled was no more encouraging about my new phase than my gynecologist's gloomy assessment. I found an unbroken litany of the supposedly inevitable scourges of menopause. On a yellow legal pad I made a list: hot flashes, night sweats, crippling osteoporosis, potential chronic heart problems, weight gain that promised thickening rolls of fat around stomach and thighs, declining libido, loss of concentration and memory difficulties, aging skin, irritability, mood swings and depression, severe headaches, sensory disturbances, dizzy spells, panic attacks, frequent urination, vaginal dryness, joint pain, lack of energy, and changes in hair quality. God, I thought, just give me a gun so I can shoot myself.

These warnings are foreboding to say the least. And because the mind can play such a strong role in our psychological makeup as well as our physical well-being, if we are constantly told that these are the "natural" effects of menopause, then no wonder almost every woman I know looks forward to this phase of her life with such dread. Now I knew why I never heard women say, "Oh, I can't wait until I get to menopause, it's going to be such a positive, life-changing experience."

But while everything I read that day was filled with stiflingly repetitive warnings, I found little or nothing on ways to combat the effects. Of course, there was the ever-present recommendation of hormone replacement therapy—cited by several books as a miracle cure. It had such allure. On one side of my legal paper, I had this long list of disturbing symptoms, and medical science was holding out the promise that a simple pill could bypass all that trouble. It was a powerful inducement in a culture where we increasingly want simple answers to complex questions.

But this first batch of books and articles left me with the same alternative I had when I left my gynecologist's office—menopause was presented as an illness. Women entering menopause have a hormone deficiency, according to the standard books, and therefore if we are given hormones the deficiency is corrected and we are "cured." Even the language chosen by the pharmaceutical companies—hormone replacement therapy—suggests that we've lost something we need to get back. And studies show that women who think of menopause as an illness are the most likely to take hormones. If you instead think of menopause as a natural transition, you're less likely to believe you need medicine to cure a problem.

One article even drew a comparison between menopause and diabetes, saying that when a person's insulin levels can't maintain normal blood sugar levels, insulin is given and the balance is reinstated. This just didn't sit right with me. Diabetes is not a natural event in our lives but rather an illness. Yet every woman will pass through menopause. No matter what I read, I wasn't going to be convinced that menopause is an illness or an affliction.

Instead, I viewed menopause as a natural progression in any woman's life, one that I expected might have some uncomfortable symptoms but that on the whole would put me on some other interesting and challenging path once I had passed through it. I had faced many stumbling blocks in life and had approached each as an obstacle that could be overcome. "Trisha, you can do this," I always told myself. This was no different. I wasn't depressed about having entered menopause early, but I was dejected at not finding anyone who presented a positive program to adjust to the upcoming effects. I wasn't looking for medication; I wanted a regimen that might help buffer the symptoms naturally while allowing me to retain all the vigor and youthfulness I had before starting.

After a couple of hours and two coffees (yes, I had read the warnings to cut down on caffeine in order to minimize possible headaches and breast tenderness, but I figured the hell with it for this first day), I shoved the stack of books to one side and left the library. That evening, at my health club, I decided to ask some of the women in their fifties about their experiences with menopause. The year before I had attended a one-day seminar on menopause at the same health club. I had clearly been the youngest woman present, and while I had gone out of mere curiosity, I had little interest in the lecturing gynecologist's exhortations about estrogen replacement. Now I sought out women I had seen at that seminar. These were women I had known as fitness mates for a couple of years, and on different occasions, while working out on stationary bikes or treadmills, we had talked about everything from world politics to Hollywood gossip. Now I approached a handful of those I knew best, confident they would help with some sage advice.

"Menopause?" the first said, looking at me somewhat quizzically. "Oh, I haven't started it yet. So I don't know what to tell you." Hmmm. That seemed strange, considering that she was in her mid-fifties. Later I learned that most women start perimenopause as early as their late thirties. But, unaware of that at the time, I let my friend off the hook with her simple denial.

The next woman I asked was only moderately more helpful. "Oh, mine was easy," she said, as she kept jogging on the treadmill. "I really didn't have any symptoms to speak of, so I guess I can't be of much help to you." I got similar responses from each of three other women I asked that evening. Even more unusual, these were acquaintances who were so talkative that other gym members sometimes complained that our lively discussions were distracting. Once started on a subject, my gym buddies were usually well informed and certainly not shy about sharing their opinions. But when it came to menopause, they were not only unenthusiastic about pursuing the conversation but quite eager to either change the subject or end our talk. I was discovering that the writer Gail Sheehy was right when she said, "Menopause may be the last taboo," and dubbed women afraid of talking about it as "monophobic."

When I got home I called one of my dearest friends, Marion, who, in her mid-sixties, must have been through menopause. She was quite willing to discuss her bout with change, and as it turned out, she was almost a poster girl for the worst of the symptoms I had read about at the library. I didn't know it at the time, but Marion would eventually be my only friend who would openly talk about her passage. She also warned me that few women would be frank and forthcoming on the topic, especially in our age-obsessed culture. "A lot of it is about age," Marion said. "Women know that menopause pegs them at a certain age, and they don't want that. Why do you think that you almost never hear Hollywood stars who are menopausal—like Susan Sarandon, Barbra Steisand, Bette Midler, and Goldie Hawn—talk about it? It would be reminding the whole world that they are in their fifties. I have girlfriends who would never disclose that they've passed menopause because somehow it makes them feel younger, or sexier, to pretend they haven't crossed into it."

I have never been bothered by age. Sure, there are things like getting by on four hours of sleep at night, or drinking a bit too much, that I can't do as well in my late forties as when I was in my late twenties. But I am so much happier, and more complete as a woman, at my current age than when I was twenty-five, I wouldn't trade it for anything. My age is a badge of achievement, an indication that I have learned something in life. Since I had never concealed my real age, I was surprised to learn that hiding the experience of menopause might be related to that unfortunate fear of aging that afflicts so many women. But Marion's words rang true. I thought of a talk show I had watched a few nights earlier on which a prominent actress had openly discussed her dysfunctional childhood, her bouts with depression, and her fight with fat, but left out of her litany of life experiences was any mention of menopause. You would think that this mid-fifties actress had somehow never heard of the word.

A dear friend of mine who is a writer for a network soap opera was not surprised when I told her about what I was discovering. "Trisha, you may not watch soaps enough to know this, but we never have any of our characters go into menopause," she said. "Oh, everything happens to them— they become alcoholics, get charged with murder, have multiple affairs, have out-of-body experiences, you name it. But not menopause. If the actress gets to that age, either she is on the other side of it without a mention or she gets replaced with someone younger. It's just not something women, who constitute the bulk of our viewers, want to see in a story line." And television isn't the only place that pretends menopause doesn't exist. In Hollywood movies it is also unheard of.

If many women are ashamed of talking about menopause because they fear it marks them as past some arbitrary prime they have set for themselves, it is little wonder that I had difficulty finding the material I needed. I had heard women discuss everything from mammograms to fitness aches and pains, but here there was little attempt to share experiences and find common ground for better alternative treatments. It reminded me of what Tina Brown, the celebrated magazine editor, had once written: "Menopause: In our youth-obsessed culture, the very word is a room-emptier." I stopped being surprised that we had allowed doctors to insert themselves into this passage as the arbiters of what we should do with our bodies. Menopause had become a secret in our closets, and we found it simpler to merely follow our doctors' advice and start on a hormone replacement program.

Following my talk with Marion, I was more convinced than ever that I was not going to go quietly into this change. I looked at the long list of "ailments" I had written down earlier at the library. These were not the markers for my menopause. I tore that sheet off the pad and marched out onto my apartment balcony. It was windy, an approaching thunderstorm due soon, but I stood there on the twenty-eighth floor, looking out toward the United Nations and the East River. With great gusto I ripped that sheet into a dozen small pieces and flung it as hard as I could into the wind. They scattered in an instant, floating out across the city. That simple act felt liberating, as though I had just tossed away my fears. Those were the things the "experts" said were inevitable. I was going to prove them wrong.

FOUR

Setting the Baseline

BEFORE settling the question of whether I would
begin hormone replacement or search for my own
program, I first had to decide which if any of the many possible symptoms I had. I sat at my dining room table and
took out another legal pad and started truthfully listing
any changes I should have noticed recently. It is easy to be
honest with a girlfriend who calls you for advice regarding
intimate parts of her life. It's not so easy sometimes to be
just as honest about the changes that you are personally undergoing. And I had to determine which I could realisti-
cally assign to menopause and which were just the results of
normal aging. Had I gained weight because my estrogen
had dropped or merely because my metabolism had slowed
as I got older? Did my skin seem less elastic and did I spot
more wrinkles because of my hormone shifts or just because

of extra years flying by? I was determined not to pull any punches.

Mood swings? Possibly. Gerald used to say that I was the happiest and most positive person he had ever met. It took a lot to put me into a bad mood, and fairly extreme behavior to make me lose my temper. But, as I thought about it, I realized that during the past six months or so I might have been edgier, quicker to take insult at a perceived slight, and faster to snap back at someone over silly matters. And more noticeable than any increased irritability were occasional bouts of feeling blue. There had been a few times when I'd suddenly turned to Gerald and confided, "I feel like bursting into tears."

"Why?" he would invariably ask.

"I don't know." That was the most frustrating aspect, not knowing why these somber moods would suddenly settle over me. And then, as unexpectedly as they had arrived, they would be gone in a few hours. I remember thinking that if this malaise became a constant cloud, it could be completely debilitating. And these blue periods stood out so clearly because they were so different from anything I had ever experienced. Sometimes I would just wake up feeling depressed, and other times, for no apparent reason, I would get into an utter gloom in the middle of the day.

Hot flashes? Yes, again, while I had tried to ignore them, there was little doubt that they had been bothering me. The symptoms of menopause vary widely from woman to woman; instead of the sleep-interrupting, body-drenching night sweats often reported in the literature, I would get a flash while awake. And no matter when they struck, my face was never involved; the heat wave just passed up my torso. It was, as I once said to Gerald, the strangest feeling, as though someone had turned on an unknown internal furnace. Even if I was in the middle of a cold air-conditioned room, this internal heat was unavoidable once it started. And there was my own strange symptom—hot feet—on some nights when I went to bed.

Sometimes of late I had been particularly fatigued. Also, problems I'd had several years earlier with digestive cramping and bloating had largely disappeared until some recent bouts. And I now recalled some moments during the past few months when my heart had seemed to race for no apparent reason, a rapid palpitation that would last no longer than a minute. I felt it was so loud that people could actually hear it. I would steady myself and take some deep breaths that would usually return it to a normal rate, but those little attacks were often frightening.

But, partly because none of these symptoms had been regular, I had ignored them, assuring myself that if they were evidence of some medical condition they would be constant. That had been, of course, just another form of denial.

What about other typical symptoms associated with menopause? Thinning hair or drying skin? Girls, for this I left the table and grabbed a magnifying mirror from the bathroom. Those mirrors are horrendous to use because they tend to make any simple hair follicle appear to be an entire beard or cast a simple blemish as a veritable volcanic eruption. But, deciding that this physical review had to be more honest than kind, I stared in the mirror as I gently tugged on my face and neck, trying to see if my skin appeared dry. I even put on my reading glasses, another sign of passing into middle age, which added a little extra magnification.

I've always had very fair skin and have moisturized it and used sunscreens for years. Now, maybe it was my imagination, but it did seem a bit drier. But this was nothing that a little extra moisturizer—at least as a temporary Band-Aid of sorts—couldn't help. My thick and curly hair, of which I have always been proud, seemed to be fine. But if I tugged on it anymore, examining the long strands, I might well cause it to thin just by pulling it out.

What of any loss of libido? I certainly thought that an active sex life was an important aspect of why our marriage was so successful. There were friends of mine who described barren relationships, and while they often got along great with their husbands, there was something important missing. Yet, as I thought more about it, we had been far less active in the last six months than ever before. We had both ascribed it to the pressures of too many deadlines and too much stress. But recently, even when Gerald was in the mood, I had found myself strangely ambivalent, invariably leading to a polite "No, this isn't the right time" answer. It wasn't that I did not want sex, but rather that I just couldn't be bothered. That was strange, but it had seemed a passing phase. Now I worried that it was a turning point that might continue and affect our marriage.

What about thickening flab around the stomach? The weight on my five-foot-seven frame varied between 127 and 132 pounds. Twelve years earlier, when I had given up smoking, I had blissfully ballooned up to 145 before being dumbstruck on a scale one day. I'd kicked the scale across the room, convinced it was lying to me. But I had slowly lost the extra pounds by changing my eating habits to those recommended by most doctors and nutritionists, high in carbohydrates and low in saturated fats. I could grab a roll of skin around my midriff, but who couldn't? My clothes still fit, so I decided I had not yet lost muscle to fat.

Memory loss? None that I could think of. But that wasn't very reassuring; I had never been that great at remembering telephone numbers or names. But at least there didn't appear to be any changes for the worse.

And while I wanted to know more about the condition of my bones and heart, I knew that would mean additional medical testing. I asked Gerald what he thought about the idea of getting some baseline tests done.

"I think it's great," he said without any hesitation. "If you don't have some real tests done, there's no way you'll know whether you are improving with your own program or whether the doctors are right and you need estrogen. Do it."

"Well, there's not much, except for a bone density test, and then I can have my cholesterol checked, and also have a stress test on a treadmill," I told him.

"And while you're at it," he said, "you might as well have one of the fitness trainers at the gym do a body fat measurement."

"Why would I want to do that?" I asked indignantly. I worked out three to five days a week, doing at least half an hour on a stationary bike or treadmill for my cardiovascular

training and then taking one of the classes, which ranged
from stretch sessions to other types of mild conditioning. I
thought I was very fit. "Are you saying I'm fat?"

"No, no, no." The slight anxiety in his voice indicated
that he knew he was treading on thin ice, weight being one
of my most sensitive subjects. "It's just, that, while, sometimes . . ."

"Get it out. Come on, stop torturing me, just tell me
what you're thinking."

"It's just that, in the last year, I think you are as fit as
ever, and your weight is great . . ."

"But?"

"But you seem somehow a little softer to me."

"Softer? What?"

"Flabbier. Not as lean."

"You're nuts." I waved him away. "Now I know you're
nuts. I weigh a hundred twenty-eight pounds, and I eat
healthy."

"I know that," he countered, knowing that he was unlikely to convince me otherwise. "But you were the one
who showed me the articles you copied from the library, the
ones that indicated there is an inevitable replacement of
muscle tissue with fat at menopause and middle age. You're
there. Don't be blind to those changes, even if they are subtle."

"Oh, sometimes I don't even know why I ask you," I dis-
missed him, as I left the room.

Some nerve. Flabby. Gerald also worked hard at staying
fit, but did he think he was Mr. America? I stopped in front

of the mirror near the kitchen and held my arms out to the side. There under each one was loose skin, and if I touched it, it moved back and forth. It was exactly what made you hide your sleeveless dresses in the back of the closet. And I didn't need to pull down my trousers to see the two bumps that had formed along the sides of my thighs. When I was a kid, my family used to feed me extra food to fatten me up because I was rail thin with sticks for legs. In my twenties and thirties, even if I temporarily gained weight, I stayed straight around my thighs. Then, in my forties, I started to develop saddlebags. It seemed as if any new weight went first to my thighs and stomach. That dreaded middle-age spread, a matronly body, something that none of us think we will get until it happens. *Flabby* might have been the wrong word—and it was pretty undiplomatic, I thought— but Gerald was only trying to be honest in this new endeavor. And although his straightforwardness could sometimes be unsettling, being utterly frank with each other was something we prized. All right, it wouldn't kill me—I would add the body fat test to my set of baselines.

Within a couple of weeks I had my results. My bone density test was good, certainly normal for a woman my age, and not showing any early warning signs of osteoporosis. Even my gynecologist was pleased, but he used the results as another opportunity to recommend that I immediately start a hormone replacement program.

"Trisha, these figures are so good that this is the time to ensure you keep them this good. You're into menopause, and if you don't take precautions now, your test results will dramatically worsen. Estrogen is the only protector you have available; the reports are clear about that."

I am nothing if not stubborn, though, and it did not take him long to realize that I was still not ready.

My stress test on a treadmill was passed easily, at a rate that my general practitioner said was more like that of someone years younger. My cholesterol was at 195, with a fine ratio of the good to bad kind.

Actually, the only disappointing news was that damn body fat exam at my gym. After carefully measuring a dozen spots with a pair of metal calipers and working out a series of calculations, the fitness trainer told me I had 34 percent body fat.

"How is that possible when I don't eat that much fat?"

"A lot of women your age"—God, how I hate that phrase—"have much higher fat," he tried to reassure me. "Much of it is just age. Our calculations change on this chart depending on age. If you are the same weight as you were twenty or thirty years earlier, you will actually have more fat since you just lose your muscle as you get older. That's why a man who weighs the same at seventy as he did at twenty could never fit into the uniform he wore as a young soldier. He would have to weigh less, and be doing exercises that would add back muscle, to get into that uniform."

I sighed. This was going to be more work than I'd expected. No wonder some women just threw up their hands and asked their doctors to write a prescription for estrogen. It was time to return to the library and the Internet and see what I could find to maintain my bone and heart results while adjusting my weight and body fat and fighting my recent symptoms, ranging from the mildly aggravating hot flashes to the more worrisome bouts of the blues. My body wasn't behaving the way I expected it to, and I was ready to go to war to make sure I put it on the path I wanted. Now I just had to figure out the right strategy.

FIVE

The Hormone Machine

ONE of the first things I had to confront was whether my fear of hormone replacement was well founded or just unreasonable, as my gynecologist had warned. It turns out that many women have the same concern. A large study a few years ago revealed that 30 percent of the women who receive a prescription for hormones never fill it, another 20 percent stop taking it in less than nine months, and another 10 percent ignore the dosage information and take it only intermittently. In the United States, where doctors have largely fallen into lockstep behind the American Medical Association's recommendation of hormone replacement, about a quarter of all menopausal women are on a prescription program. And although they aren't experts on heart disease or osteoporosis, the two big illnesses for which hormones are most often touted, American gynecologists are now responsible for most of the hormone prescriptions written each year. In Europe, where doctors aren't so estrogen gung-ho, only 3 to 4 percent of all menopausal women use hormone replacement therapy. There, 30 to 40 percent of doctors rely on herbal remedies as their primary treatment.

After a week of plowing through books and articles, I felt better about deciding not to accept my gynecologist's advice so readily. I did find evidence that his strident view was not unique, at least in the United States. As early as the 1950s, a few doctors had begun classifying menopause as "estrogen deficiency" disease, an affliction that needed medication for treatment. One book I came across, *Feminine Forever,* was written in 1966 by a New York gynecologist, Robert Wilson. He really got my blood going, especially when he drew ridiculous conclusions like "The unpalatable truth must be faced that all postmenopausal women are castrates. . . . From a practical point of view, a man remains a man until the very end. The situation with a woman is very different. Her ovaries become inadequate relatively early in life. She is the only mammal who cannot reproduce after middle age."

Wilson had zeroed in on the fact that healthy menopausal women have plenty of hormones for everything but childbearing. A hundred years ago the average woman didn't live past her reproductive years. Now that we live longer lives, doctors like Wilson denigrated us as somehow less than complete because of a change that nature programmed into our biological makeup. His description of his mother's menopause was of a terrible affliction: "I was appalled at the transformation of that vital, wonderful woman who had been the dynamic focal point of our family into a pain-racked petulant invalid. I could feel the deep wounds her senseless rages inflicted on my father, myself, and the younger children. It was this frightful experience that later directed my interest as a physician to the problem of menopause."

Wilson's bestselling book, backed financially by the medical lab that produced the most widely prescribed estrogen replacement, had a major impact in the 1960s, almost single-handedly establishing the notion that, since estrogen-starved women were a misery to themselves and society in general, estrogen replacement was heaven-sent. As a result of his work, most doctors accepted that menopause was a treatable medical condition. Hormones replaced the tranquilizers and antidepressants that had been promoted by American physicians in the 1950s and early 1960s to "cure" menopausal symptoms. I found it rather amusing that before Wilson's work we were told that menopausal symptoms were in our heads, and therefore treated as though we had a psychiatric problem. After Wilson the symptoms were suddenly acknowledged as real, and we were all supposed to treat them with a wonder drug. In overblown prose Wilson told women that estrogen replacement was "a precious gift" and promised that by taking hormones we would achieve "final emancipation." Without estrogen, he warned, we were destined to become sexless "caricatures of [our] former selves . . . the equivalent of a eunuch."

Wilson described his examination of a fifty-two-year-old woman on hormones and how startled he was at her youthful appearance. "I therefore believe," he wrote, "that menopause prevention far transcends the purely clinical aspects of the subject. It even transcends any narrow view of sex as such. What is really at stake is a subtle and almost metaphysical factor—a woman's total femininity." Wilson masterfully played off women's fears about aging. Although his language now seems remarkably anachronistic, his argument for hormone replacement could be powerfully seductive in our youth-obsessed culture. Just at the point when menopause screams to us "middle age," serving as an intrusive reminder that our youth is quickly fading, Wilson held out the promise that it could all go away with a little pill.

I noticed that while I was reading this book a young man who had been sitting at the same library table gathered his books and moved one table away. I guess that as my anger slowly built, a deep scowl had appeared on my face and virtual steam came from my ears.

I did relax considerably when I later read that many Asian cultures have much more refreshing views of menopause. They consider it a critically important phase of a woman's life, actually slowing the aging process so the body can flourish for decades longer. I knew that while my body was going through changes, it certainly was not burdened with a disease, and if somebody called me a "castrate" he would get more than a piece of my mind.

My original fear about hormone replacement had been focused on breast cancer and my family history. But I soon discovered considerable safety concerns over many aspects of synthetic hormones. Side effects such as water retention and bloating, tender breasts, headaches, and weight gain were upsetting but not serious. Others were more bothersome, including depression, increased susceptibility to vaginal yeast infections, skin rashes, hair loss, abdominal cramps, nausea, changes in libido, increased blood pressure, and cystitislike syndromes. Side effects that might be life threatening, including stroke and pulmonary thrombophlebitis (a dangerous inflammation of the veins), are still subjects of heated disagreement within the medical community.

Synthetic estrogen is almost never prescribed alone, because there is no doubt that it dramatically boosts the odds of uterine cancer, up to thirteen times greater risk than for a woman not on the hormone. Since the late 1970s, when doctors discovered this risk and the FDA issued a warning about it, prescriptions have commonly been mixed with some progestin, a synthetic version of the natural hormone progesterone that provides some protection against uterine cancer. But I quickly discovered that progestins often induce a wide range of side effects, most of which mimic the worst of those in menopause. Many women who start a program of hormone replacement have to stop in less than a year because of depression, bloating, irritability, abdominal cramps, headaches, and hot flashes. A majority drop off the program within two years, finding the side effects more bothersome than their original menopausal discomforts. And progestin also induces uterine bleeding, meaning that, as long as you use it, you have an unnatural "period." Worsened symptoms were certainly not what I was looking for.

As for my specific concern—increased risk of breast cancer—I was surprised to learn that the largest study measur-

ing the long-term effects of an estrogen-progesterone therapy—undertaken by the National Institutes of Health and
the Women's Health Institute—will not be finished until
between 2005 and 2008. It seemed a little premature for
me to rush into a medical treatment that might have to be
a lifelong commitment before the definitive data on its
safety are available.

Although the debate over estrogen and breast cancer
seems to change depending on the latest study, in June
1999 the *Journal of the American Medical Association* published the results of a ten-year study of 37,105 menopausal
women. As for any study that shows a benefit from hormone therapy, the drug companies went into high gear to
assure it received lots of media attention. The results were
touted by much of the press as definitive proof that there
was little if any link between estrogen replacement therapy
and breast cancer. "A Study Plays Down Estrogen Link to
Breast Cancers" was the *New York Times* headline. (By that
time, I was far along on my own program that eschewed estrogen, but still I read the results carefully to see whether
my initial fears had been overblown.)

When I read beyond the headline, I discovered that the
study wasn't quite what was being promoted. It did show
that the most common types of breast cancers were not increased by estrogen. However, women who took hormones
had greater incidences of three types of breast cancer that
tend to be stimulated by—no surprise here—estrogen. The
doctors behind the study tried to minimize these results by
emphasizing that the breast cancers caused by estrogen re-
spond well to treatment and are less likely than other tu-

mors to spread. Well, easy-to-cure cancer or not, no thanks. If those are considered good odds, with my family history, that study only confirmed my satisfaction in having passed.

Even that highly touted result was contradicted by a review by British doctors, who combined data from more than fifty major studies. They flatly concluded that the longer a woman took hormones, the greater her risk of breast cancer. There was about a 35 percent increased risk if you were on hormones for five or fewer years. That seemed really high to me. After five years the odds of developing breast cancer were even worse, and the mortality rate started climbing.

I did notice that some new studies promoted so-called designer estrogens, such as raloxifene and tamoxifen, as wonder drugs without increased breast cancer odds. In fact, tamoxifen is given to some women diagnosed with breast cancer. Both my mother and my aunt had been treated with it after their breast cancer diagnoses. In many articles these new estrogens are described as cure-alls without side effects. But a little extra research reconfirmed that there is no free lunch. Not only do the designer estrogens do little to alleviate the symptoms of menopause—and may in some cases, like hot flashes, actually exacerbate them—but they bring along their own risks, ranging from cosmetic disasters like alopecia (total hair loss) through more serious problems like vision impairment to potentially fatal side effects like blood clots. Tamoxifen, after prolonged use, can actually cause some other types of cancers. Once again, massive studies that might provide some long-term answers are under way; the results should be ready about

2004. Until then, no thanks. I just don't like being an unpaid guinea pig for large pharmaceutical companies that are trying hard to develop effective (and profitable) treatments.

The final wrinkle I came across early in my research was the trend among some doctors to add the male hormone testosterone to the drug regimen for menopausal women. Touted as a natural antidepressant, testosterone has become an increasingly popular add-on for hormone replacement therapy in the hope that it will combat the blues and loss of sexual appetite many women experience. But I'm surprised that any postmenopausal woman who has read about the side effects would willingly take this hormone. All women naturally produce testosterone. Before menopause, estrogen keeps its side effects in check. After menopause, with the testosterone in the body unchecked by estrogen, some women find that their voices deepen and in rare cases develop facial or chest hair. Giving women the hormone enhances the odds of these effects. These changes may *not* be reversible. If that's not bad enough, testosterone also causes a lot of women to gain weight. Now, if I took testosterone to alleviate the blahs, I can't imagine something that would make me feel bluer than having to pluck hairs from my face daily and have my chest waxed so I could wear a T-shirt without hair showing. Again, if that was the best that science was offering, it was not right for me.

"Well, I certainly made the right decision in passing on hormones," I announced with satisfaction to Gerald when I walked into the apartment. "There's just no definitive data about whether they are safe for the long term."

"So where does that leave you?" he asked.

"That's what I'm trying to figure out. Now I'm getting into uncharted waters."

The challenge before me was daunting but also straight-forward. On one side of a sheet of paper I had listed the benefits touted by medical science in favor of hormone replacement. Among them was promised relief from meno-pausal symptoms such as night sweats, hot flashes, loss of sexual desire, depression, and memory loss. Estrogen also supposedly helps battle some of the aging effects of meno-pause, like drying skin and thinning hair. Some other ben-efits were important but limited. Hormones assist a woman's bones and might guard against osteoporosis. An-other major benefit touted by many doctors is protection against the onset of heart disease. Since far more women die from heart ailments than from breast cancer, this is consid-ered one of the strongest advantages to a program of hor-mones, although one major 1985 study showed that the risk of heart disease *increased* for women taking hormones. And the major study cited to show that estrogen helps the heart was done on men only!

On the other side of the paper I had a lot of blank spaces. Now I needed to fill in those blanks with the names of nat-ural remedies and therapies that might achieve the same re-sults. I wanted all the benefits without the hormones. I wanted to discover choices I never knew I had. Soon I would know if that was possible.

SIX

Estrogen Is Estrogen

AT my local health food store I spent so long huddled in the small corner where the books were kept that the manager came by several times to make sure I had not converted his tiny storefront into a lending library. I was skimming through a score of books that promised natural alternatives for dealing with menopause, trying to narrow my choices down to a dozen or so. Although they seemed to offer a grab bag of generalizations together with almost overwhelming lists of herbal and natural remedies, I hoped to use them as a starting point for fashioning a trial-and-error approach for my symptoms. When I finally deposited my basket of books in front of the cashier, a woman who was walking past glanced over.

"Somebody you know going through menopause?" she asked. She seemed to be slightly older than me.

"Yes. Me."

"Oh, my," she said, looking genuinely surprised. "You seem too young."

"Thank you," I replied. "I want to stay that way, hence the books."

"Interesting" was all she said as she walked away.

When I left the store, I noticed she was now in the front corner, flipping through some of the same books I had been looking at. Maybe women only need a little encouragement, I thought, to start researching the possibilities beyond hormone replacement.

At home I curled up on the sofa, spread the books across the coffee table, and began reading. With only a short break for dinner, by midnight I had skimmed through nearly all of them. The following day, with the books stuffed with bright yellow Post-it notes and marked all along the margins with my trademark purple ballpoint pen, I settled in front of the computer and logged on to the Internet to find even more information about those herbs, vitamins, and lifestyle changes that seemed intriguing. As that day drew to a close, I had nearly a thousand pages of printouts from articles and studies.

"That's why women take hormones," Gerald said as he looked at the growing piles of paper. "It's a hell of a lot simpler to take that pill every day than to go through this."

"Sure, but I like the research, you know that."

"I understand, but most women don't have the same inclination or the time," he said.

"You might only have to do this once," I said, glancing at the paperwork. "Once you know what really works and what doesn't, you never have to do it again. This is the groundwork for finding the program that will really work."

He smiled. "That's why I first fell in love with you. You never think small."

One of the reasons I knew any successful natural program would take a lot of work was that all of my symptoms might not be the result of a shortage of hormones. Although doctors tend to lump together all the symptoms I had been experiencing as menopausal, many could have been the result of other problems, ranging from nutritional imbalances to the incorrect mixture of supplements and vitamins. A complete program through menopause would have to involve some balancing of my hormones, a change in my diet, a new exercise routine, a modified beauty regimen, and a menu of mineral, vitamin, and herb supplements. And I had made the challenge even greater by deciding to do all this without the benefit of advice from my gynecologist or general practitioner. Normally, I think you should always ask your doctor before fiddling around with your body and what you put in it. But I already knew that in this instance my doctors didn't have the answers for which I was searching. I would not only have to carefully monitor the side effects and long-term health risks of the treatments I chose, but I would also have to determine how those treatments worked with one another. By cutting out my doctors, I was ensuring a lot of extra work and responsibility on my end. It was exhausting just to contemplate.

One possible shortcut was something I came across in my first major blast of research—the so-called natural hormones. All of these promised relief from aggravating symptoms, plus bone and heart benefits, and none of the risks of synthetic hormones. So I trekked out during a particularly nasty downpour to a nearby health food store. I wanted to see these products firsthand. As I stood dripping all over the front of the store, one of the clerks, looking a bit like Woody Allen but with a curly mop of hair that could have used a good washing, hovered nearby. When he asked if I needed any help, I told him I was looking for the section with herbs and vitamins related to menopause. No sooner had I gotten the words out than he scurried down an aisle, exhorting me to follow him. He stopped, grabbed a jar off a shelf, and whirled around to face me.

"This is all you'll need," he said triumphantly, as though he had been waiting all day for someone to ask him this one question.

"What is it?"

"We call it 'Miracle in a Jar,'" he said. Already I was suspicious. "It's made from yams, and it provides natural estrogen and progesterone. This is exactly what you're missing when you enter menopause. Is this for someone you know?"

"It might be for me."

"Hmmm," he mumbled as he stared at me, trying to figure out whether I was doing some advance research or was in menopause now. Evidently satisfying himself, he continued. "Well, these hormones—"

"But I've decided not to use hormones, I'm looking—"

My helpful clerk waved away my remarks with a sweeping gesture. "No, no, no. These are *natural*." He emphasized the word as though it were a magic talisman. "They are just like the hormones in your body," he continued, "and they carry none of the risks associated with synthetic hormones. We have many, many satisfied customers. And since no big drug companies are behind these, pushing up the prices, it's not expensive—only thirty-five dollars a jar, and it should last for weeks. Will you try one?"

He had to be kidding. I had been refusing to listen to the advice of my trusted gynecologist, who at least had been through medical school, and this store clerk thought I was going to rely on his thirty-second pitch?

"It sounds very interesting, but I'd like some more information first," I replied. "Do you have any pamphlets about it that I could take with me?"

"Oh, instructions come with the cream, and they explain a lot."

"No. I need more information than a product insert." Beating around the bush wasn't getting me far, so it was time to be more direct. "I'll pass for now."

He seemed crestfallen. I'm still not sure whether he took my no as a personal rejection of his judgment, or if I had somehow wandered into the only vitamin store in New York City where the staff was on commission. I almost ran from the shop.

While that clerk may not have made a sale, he did focus me even more on the relatively new and increasingly popular trend toward "natural," plant-derived hormone replacements, such as those found in wild yam and soy products. I decided that the next phase of my research would be trying to determine whether these products would be right for me.

It did not take very long to discover that many women, as the clerk had claimed, have been attracted to these plant compounds, usually called "the naturals." Yet, despite their name, the hormones found in these products, including estrogen, progesterone, and testosterone, are created in laboratories. They are called natural only because they are biologically identical to human hormones.

The chemist who discovered the ability to convert certain plant by-products into hormones, in the 1930s, never patented his discovery. As a result, for many years no U.S. drug company aggressively pursued the natural compounds, since they could not reap the profits the way they can when they develop and patent a laboratory-designed synthetic from the ground up. In an era of considerable mistrust of pharmaceutical companies and a widespread belief that they sometimes place our well-being below the goal of earning high profits, the very fact that the largest conglomerates have not produced plant-derived hormones enhances the attraction of these compounds for many women.

Some of the literature I found contended that the plant-derived hormones must be better for us since they come from nature. This certainly sounds plausible when you consider that Premarin—with a billion dollars a year in sales, the most widely prescribed prescription drug in the United States—comes from the urine of pregnant horses (the trade name is shorthand for "pregnant mare's urine"). Premarin had been widely popular in the 1970s, with almost 30 million annual prescriptions. Then the news that estrogen led to uterine cancer caused its popularity to plummet. But the drug was saved from extinction when doctors discovered that by mixing in some progesterone the endometrial cancer risk was greatly reduced. By the mid-1990s, with drug companies finding new ways to promote estrogen replacement as a "necessity," Premarin approached 50 million annual prescriptions. Somehow, at least to me, plant-derived estrogen identical to that in my body did seem a little safer than horse estrogen.

Some, like Dr. John Lee, the author of the popular 1996 book *What Your Doctor May Not Tell You About Menopause,* contended that natural progesterone alone not only alleviated the undesirable symptoms of menopause but had far fewer unpleasant side effects than completely synthetic hormones. As a result of Lee's recommendation and those of other prominent advocates, many middle-aged women in America and Europe use a progesterone cream, Pro-Gest, sold by health food stores, mail-order companies, and Internet sites. It promises, as do similar creams, to alleviate hot flashes while preserving bone density, with virtually no side effects.

However, I was not so easily sold on the naturals. True, they came from plants, and a few large drug companies were pushing them. But I was worried that by choosing them I was following the same path—hormone replacement—suggested by my gynecologist, just under a different name. And after a little reading, I discovered some more fundamental worries. The amounts of estrogen and progesterone in yam creams and the like are difficult to measure. Some of the natural products tested by labs contained no hormones at all, making them expensive but essentially useless skin creams, while other products had high levels.

Because the Food and Drug Administration won't allow the manufacturers of the creams to make medical claims, they are sold as cosmetics, which are unregulated, rather than hormone replacements. Nowhere on their labels is the word *progesterone.* They are advertised only as "wild yam extracts" or "moisturizing creams."

Even the basic question of whether hormones can be effectively administered through a topical cream is unanswered. Studies contradict one another. Some American reviews claim that natural progesterone, like that found in Pro-Gest, is readily absorbed into the skin, but they acknowledge that this is a very difficult way to achieve normal and consistent levels of the hormone. But two recent British studies concluded that natural progesterone is not properly absorbed through the skin and that, to have even the slightest results, massive quantities would have to be used. A Belgian study showed that the creams tend to accumulate in the skin instead of being absorbed into the bloodstream.

Moreover, whatever progesterone gets past the skin apparently turns up in great concentrations in the saliva but not in the uterus, where it might protect against cancer, and not in the bones, where it might help fight osteoporosis. And some women, sensitive to progesterone, experience the same aggravating symptoms associated with premenstrual syndrome or menopause itself. Others report being constantly tired, light-headed, or dizzy, and suffering from tender breasts, increased light sensitivity in their eyes, and skin problems such as acne. Progesterone can also increase the risk of heart disease by decreasing the level of good cholesterol in our bodies. With such dismal results, I certainly could find better ways to spend my money than on a thirty-five-dollar jar of Pro-Gest or a similar progesterone cream.

Once again it seemed to me that the proponents of so-called natural hormones had jumped the gun. One larger study under way in Britain may answer some of these questions, but it won't have results for a few more years. The jury is still out on not only the possible benefits of the naturals but also whether they are effective at all. It seemed silly to so stridently say no to my doctor's advice to start a program of hormone replacement and then adopt my own program with over-the-counter hormones from a local health food store. The theory behind natural progesterone is really the same as the theory behind regular hormone replacement therapy: Women are suffering from a hormone deficiency disorder, and the creams can help correct our imbalance.

I wanted to develop an entirely different approach. Like the purveyors of hormones, I wanted to battle the symptoms of menopause, protect my heart, keep my cancer risks low, and improve my appearance. My early reading had convinced me that I wanted to find a program that was completely hormone-free. There was, I quickly learned, no shortcut.

SEVEN

"Is It Hot in Here?"

SOME episodes during menopause stand out. Most of them revolve around hot flashes. A typical one occurred when I was out for dinner with Gerald and a group of friends. It was a Friday evening, the end of a particularly hectic week. It felt great to be away from deadlines and relax. I had just started to scan the menu, trying to find a dish not swamped in butter or cream, when I felt that familiar sensation of warmth somewhere near my stomach. Then a wave of heat started filling my chest. It was as though I had a radiator in my body, and suddenly it was flipped on and set to high. The dining room quickly seemed stifling.

"Is it hot in here, or is it me?" I whispered to Gerald.

"It's you," he said quietly, a knowing look of sympathy etched on his face.

Gently I closed my menu and started fanning myself. My

friends knew I'd been flirting with menopause. They all did their best to pretend nothing was out of the ordinary, despite the fact that I was waving an oversized menu in front of my face in a perfectly climate-controlled room.

On another occasion, at another restaurant, the heat became so unbearable that I asked the waiter for a glass of ice water and guzzled it. No help. Then I retreated to the ladies' room with a few cubes of ice and rubbed them vigorously behind my ears and on my wrists, a trick my mother had taught me as a youngster to cool off during rare British heat waves. Besides earning the bewildered stare of the bathroom attendant, the ice managed only to make my ears and wrists cold.

Around the time I began researching alternatives to hormone replacement therapy, I was minding my own business in an office supplies store when I suddenly felt an intense wave of heat. Gerald was with me as I took my wool overcoat off and dragged it along the floor behind me as I slouched uncomfortably around the aisles, looking in vain for some pocket of the store where I might get an unblocked stream of air-conditioning.

"I feel like ripping my clothes off," I muttered to myself, angry that my body was betraying me this way. Peeling off clothes—just short of removing the layer that might lead to my arrest for indecent exposure—was one of my natural reactions to the more severe attacks. One of the young store clerks must have overheard me, because he suddenly seemed to be everywhere I went in the store. The poor chap must have interpreted my frustration as a real promise to disrobe.

Ah, hot flashes. Unpleasant. Unexpected. And always at the worst possible times. Why didn't they come and go when I was sleeping, instead of when I was out trying to socialize and look halfway decent? No wonder irritability is one of the symptoms of menopause—few things can put you in a bad mood as quickly as having to fret over these heat attacks. They quickly take away your confidence, leaving you feeling unattractive and, especially if you are in a business setting, thinking everyone is aware of your discomfort.

I had heard about hot flashes from my mother and her friends, and when I was a teenager they seemed a funny and strange middle-age rite of passage. But now that they were happening to me, I didn't see the humor at all. I'm not sure what I expected, but it was different from anything I had imagined. Since the heat was isolated in my torso, at least my face was spared the blotchy red marks that afflict many menopausal women. I would, however, instantly start perspiring. That's always a nice touch if you're wearing something like a silk camisole.

Hot flashes are the most commonly reported menopausal symptom, with some studies showing that up to 90 percent of us have at least one, and some women actually experience them for over a decade. The few who miss this symptom should appreciate their good fortune. I realize that some women have tried to convert hot flashes into a positive experience by dubbing them "power surges." Two to 3 percent of the women in one study actually liked them. Now, I am as optimistic as the next person, and certainly capable of dealing with an unpleasant experience by trying to find something positive in it, but this seems to be pushing things just a tad. Getting to like hot flashes, at least for me, would be like embracing migraines as "tension relievers."

Since discovering that I was in full menopause, I had paid much closer attention to these flashes. I tried to determine whether there was any pattern to them, whether a certain food, drink, stress, or activity kicked them off. I kept a "hot flash diary." Caffeine, spicy foods, and alcohol were high on my list as possible triggers. But I was soon disappointed to discover there was no common thread.

And unpredictability was one of their most frustrating aspects. Sometimes they would happen when I was home alone with Gerald, but most occurred when I was out. I'll never again look askance at a middle-aged woman at the theater energetically waving her playbill in front of her face in the middle of a long second act.

"Is it hot in here?" became almost a running joke between Gerald and me. Once in a great while he would look relieved and announce somewhat enthusiastically that it was indeed hot. Then I would feel better. But most of the time he just gave me a sympathetic smile that confirmed I was having another hot flash.

Because hot flashes are such an identifiable symptom, I decided to tackle them first. My flashes had become more intense and regular over a couple of months, and I could not imagine living with this for a few years. It would be fairly easy to tell whether any natural remedy worked—the flashes would either stay or disappear. That seemed simple enough.

But *simple* and *menopause* aren't words that often fit together. I soon found out that there are many herbs and vitamins touted as cure-alls for hot flashes. If I tried several at once and the hot flashes disappeared, I would not know which did the trick. So I had to decide which sounded the most promising and offered the simplest treatment with the fewest possible side effects.

Some of the literature I read suggested only common-sense lifestyle changes to eliminate hot flashes. These included reducing stress and getting regular exercise. Since I consider these two good tenets of everyday living, I did not view them as new alternative treatments. Other suggestions, such as wearing fewer clothes or staying in very cool environments, seemed like working at the symptoms without getting at the root of the problem. A few books suggested the ancient Chinese therapy acupuncture. I had used acupuncture occasionally over the years to treat muscle and ligament injuries but just felt it was not the way I wanted to treat menopause, at least not until I had tried other routes. For instance, I was intrigued that in Japan there seem to be fewer menopausal symptoms (in the Japanese language there are not even words for "hot flash"). While I could adopt some of the elements of the Japanese diet, such as more soy-based foods and lots of fish, it seemed I would need a longer-term answer since my body had been through forty-six years of a pretty crummy Western diet.

A friend who knew of my quest suggested Bellergal, a nonhormonal drug that had helped her a decade earlier. But I did a little research and soon concluded it was not for me. Bellergal is a combination of belladonna alkaloids, ergotamine (which constricts blood vessels and is used to treat

migraines), and the barbiturate phenobarbital. It's not sur-
prising that it helps relieve hot flashes. With the powerful
sedative effect of phenobarbital, even if it didn't actually
stop the hot flashes, it would probably make you stop car-
ing about them. A potentially addictive barbiturate was
not my idea of a natural alternative to hormone replacement therapy.

Homeopathy—which involves the use of minute doses
of a remedy that would in healthy persons produce symptoms of the disease—was another suggestion in some jour-
nals. I had tried homeopathic remedies in the past, to little
avail. While I realize they are increasingly popular, especially in my native England, I could find no controlled
studies that showed homeopathic remedies might really alleviate hot flashes. And the one remedy suggested more
than any other was belladonna, a poisonous herb that is
converted to a medication for relieving spasms. It sounded
a little too serious for my taste.

Instead, I zeroed in on a group of herbs and vitamins, although I knew that just because something is an herb or vitamin doesn't mean you can't harm yourself by taking too
much of it. As you might already be able to tell, I wasn't
just going to start popping pills because some books listed
them as being good for you.

A few possibilities were quickly eliminated. For instance, a number of herbalists suggested motherwort, usually taken in a bitter liquid several times a day. Some
women swear by it, but I did not like the fact that it has
estrogen-type effects, inducing in some women heavy menstrual bleeding and, according to at least one report, stim-

ulating pregnancy-dependent breast cancers. That alone
was enough to nix it for me.

Other herbalists recommended garden sage and promoted
it for night sweats, headaches, mood swings, digestive problems, and excessive sweating. It sounded impressive. But
once again, I could not find a scientific study that related it
to menopause. Moreover, like many plants, sage also acts as a
weak estrogen. In one study it increased estrogen levels in
rats, a sure sign that women with a history of breast cancer
should avoid it. On top of this snag, I learned that too much
sage can harm both the kidneys and the liver. My hot flashes
were annoying, but nowhere near the point where I would
put the rest of my body at risk.

Black cohosh, a member of the buttercup family, seemed
far more promising. Not only had this herb been used by
Native Americans and colonists to treat menopausal symptoms, but in the twentieth century it had become a popular
alternative to estrogen replacement in parts of Europe, especially Germany. And it turned out to be the only herb on
which there were a number of controlled scientific studies,
all with promising results. For instance, in one double-
blind German study, eighty women were split into three
groups. Over twelve weeks, one group received a capsule of
black cohosh, one got the synthetic hormone Premarin, and
the last was given a placebo. The women who took black
cohosh reduced their menopausal symptoms as much as
those on Premarin did. Both of those groups did far better
than the placebo group.

Researchers have isolated one of black cohosh's effects
as decreasing the hormone levels that contribute to hot

flashes. Also, the herb might help reduce water retention, improve digestion, calm the nerves, and strengthen pelvic muscles. As with almost any drug or herb, there are side effects, but in this case they were widely reported as possible headaches or nausea. These side effects appear on the labels of most over-the-counter medicines, from flu medications to antacids. Most important for me, at least one study in mice and rats showed no estrogenic effect from black cohosh, suggesting it's safe even for women with breast cancer, not to mention for those of us who just fear getting it. Since long-term studies of its safety have not been done, a German regulatory commission suggests that black cohosh be used for no more than six months at a time. With that in mind, it was the first herb that passed my screening process. I soon had a bottle of the dry extract, 250-milligram pills, set aside in my kitchen in what was to become my growing corner for remedies.

At virtually the same time I stumbled across black cohosh, I began zeroing in on vitamin E as a potential answer to my flashes. That vitamin E was mentioned as a possible aid was and was not a surprise. I had never heard of it for this symptom, but I was used to seeing it touted as a wonder supplement for a myriad of ailments from heart disease to bad skin. Although I believe vitamin E is a marvel, and at the time I was taking 400 international units (IU) in a daily capsule, I was initially skeptical that one of its advantages could be in treating hot flashes. But after a little research I started changing my mind. One 1940s study had shown vitamin E no more effective than a placebo in treating a dozen menopausal symptoms, but it did not focus specifically on hot flashes. And many other surveys of women who had tried vitamin E as a remedy consistently showed that nearly a third considered it effective. I figured I would give it a go and doubled my daily intake to a recommended 800 IU.

Within two weeks of my taking increased amounts of vitamin E and the black cohosh, the hot flashes began abating. They dropped from nearly one or more a day to every other day, and then every third. After another two weeks my hot flashes had stopped. I had almost forgotten them. I kept thinking that it was a trick, that at any moment that heater in my body would be turned on. But it didn't happen.

I felt like a kid in a candy store. I had been diligent in finding comparatively simple and safe remedies for one of my most annoying symptoms, and it had worked. Somewhere deep down I must have had doubts about my ability to pull this off. But the hot flashes stopping so quickly emboldened me to pursue my other symptoms, as well as bolster my body in the face of the effects of entering menopause.

At the time I did not know if the ceasing of my hot flashes was permanent or not. But the more time went by without one, the more confident I became. At one point, after being clear for several months, I decided to try a small experiment to confirm that it was the right combination of vitamin E and black cohosh that had worked. I decided to slash my E intake from 800 to 400 IU while keeping the black cohosh levels the same. I dropped my vitamin E about a week before going to a lavish Thanksgiving dinner.

Gerald and I arrived at our friend's West Side apartment

in the early evening. About fifteen people were there. Somewhat nervous about the possibility of a hot flash, I wore only a skirt and silk camisole on that cool day. For a couple of hours everything seemed fine. Then, in the middle of a rather intense conversation about gun control, I felt that strange sensation kick off in my abdomen. Oh, no, I thought, it can't be. It better not be! But it was. The heat started building with an intensity I didn't remember experiencing beforehand. Hot flash free for months, I had obviously forgotten how terrible a sensation it was. Like a billowing cloud of steam, it traveled up my chest and stopped around my shoulders.

What was I to do? I looked around the apartment. I couldn't very well ask for the windows to be flung open or the air-conditioning turned on in late November. And I didn't feel it was the time or place to announce that I was in the middle of a hot flash. But I was so damn hot, I once again wanted to rip off my clothes. It was a wonder that no one noticed I was flushed.

Quickly, I excused myself and walked into the kitchen, where Neil, our host, was talking to two friends. Ignoring them, I marched directly across the room, grabbed the handle of the refrigerator door, and swung it wide. No, no, I thought. The fridge won't do. I need colder. Closing the fridge, I yanked the freezer door open so hard that a pint of ice cream flew from the door's shelf. I virtually stuffed my face inside. Ah, instant relief.

Gerald, who saw the distress on my face when I stormed toward the kitchen, had followed me. Later he told me what transpired while my head was in the freezer.

"What is she doing?" one of the girls whispered to Neil.

Neil, who knew I was going through menopause, looked over as though he could barely afford to be bothered with such a frivolous question. "Oh, her? Trisha just has a thing about freezers." Then he spun around and walked out of the kitchen. His other guests, still looking quizzically at me, followed him.

My little experiment was over. One freezer episode was enough to send me back to 800 IU of vitamin E that very night. Less than forty-eight hours later, I was again hot flash free. I haven't had one since.

EIGHT

Bonfire of the Tampons

I T was not long after starting my research, and in the middle of my work on natural progesterone, that my periods stopped completely. They had certainly been irregular, and shorter, for some time. And, as do many women, I had occasionally missed a period during the past few years, but this was the first since being told I was in menopause. The second month passed and again no period. By the third I knew this was not a fluke.

It was very strange. Instead of being sad or somehow upset, I actually felt free. Yes, of course, I was accustomed to that normal monthly ritual, but I did not always appreciate the things that went along with it, including the occasional cramping, bloating, tender breasts, several pounds of weight gain, and sometimes headaches. As a girl I had been problem free around my periods, but in my midthirties I began developing many of the menstrual symptoms my girlfriends often complained about.

"God is a man," I had confidently told my husband during one bad period.

"Why do you say that?"

"If God were a woman, men would have periods."

Even Gerald thought it made sense.

But it wasn't just the physical part that I was glad to have behind me. I was thrilled to dump the psychological baggage society attaches to a woman's monthly cycle. Premenstrual syndrome, PMS, is probably one of the most aggravating conditions medical science has isolated. To varying degrees, most women, including me, have suffered from some symptoms around our periods. A few are afflicted with really debilitating complaints. However, my objection to the increased discussion of PMS is the way that men (sorry, fellas) often use it as a weapon against us. Even my dear husband, normally a model of political correctness and sensitivity, had sometimes crossed the line.

"You're PMSing," he might blurt out in the middle of a heated disagreement. Now, that had nothing to do with which one of us was right or wrong; it was a way to let me know that I was supposedly acting badly because my body and mind were in the throes of this monthly affliction. Of course, that charge would really get me angry. That only prompted him to say, "See, you're not normally like this." Once when I was in the middle of my cycle—so I could not be charged with having PMS—I sat down with Gerald and had a long discussion about why I thought using PMS as a weapon against women was wrong. He listened and was initially somewhat defensive. But after a while, to his credit, he came around. He understood what I was saying, and why it was a sensitive issue. After that talk, he also became attuned to others using PMS in an attack mode. Often he would return from business meetings and regale me with stories of men who complained bitterly about a female supervisor's or co-worker's problems with PMS.

Now, at last, I was past it. I was into menopause, another area where men charge that women behave badly because their hormones are out of whack, but at least I was working on that and it would soon pass.

Another liberating feature of stopping my periods was that I did not have that feeling some women do of having lost their sexuality or femininity. A handful of my older friends who passed menopause several years ago told me they felt that as long as they had their periods, they were sexually attractive to men. Once they stopped, they felt as if men could sense it, knowing that these women were no longer able to bear children and therefore finding them unattractive. "A man can feel when you're no longer menstruating," one friend told me. "They have a sixth sense that you are no longer sexually interesting." Another friend was so bothered by this possibility that she even kept a box of tampons in her bathroom. She had had no reason to use them for several years but figured that if houseguests saw them they would believe she still had not entered menopause.

This was just not something that bothered me. I was in a phase where sex wasn't important to me (more about that later), but I certainly didn't feel any less sexy or attractive to men. If anything, knowing that it was unlikely I could get pregnant (there is always a chance of a pregnancy—so-called change-of-life babies—in the early stages of meno-pause) could make sex much more spontaneous than having to worry about condoms, our form of birth control for over a decade. I also had never felt as though my identity as a woman was complete only if I had children, so I did not mourn being past that stage.

It might sound strange, and it was certainly not a reac-tion I expected, but I felt liberated once I knew my periods were history.

As luck would have it, just before I was told I was menopausal, Gerald and I had taken a weekend drive to one of those huge suburban wholesale clubs. As do many city dwellers who are overwhelmed by the great discounts and enormous selection, we temporarily forgot how small our apartment was and stuffed the car to overflowing with far too many purchases. Included in that haul were several giant boxes of tampons, enough to carry me for half a year or more. Now they were stacked next to the sink in the bathroom, mocking my foolishness in stocking up as though a run on tampons was imminent.

When I told Gerald it appeared I was really done with my period, and how I felt, he understood exactly. "Con-gratulations" was his first word. His ability to often say precisely the right thing is one of the qualities I most love about him, and I could not have hoped for better than that single word.

Then I reminded him about all the tampons we had recently bought, expecting him to grimace in disapproval, since he often chides me for overstocking. The receipts were long ago thrown away, so we couldn't return them. And they aren't the types of things you give girlfriends as gifts. There was, of course, the easy route of tossing them into the garbage room. But Gerald had a better idea. "Let's have a celebration," he said. He wouldn't tell me what he had in mind, but when he is determined to do something, it is tough to dissuade him.

Two days later we packed an overnight bag; he told me we were going to a hotel for the night. I watched with amusement as he energetically stuffed all the tampons into a separate suitcase.

"What the hell are you up to?"

"Just wait and see," he said with a devilish grin. "You'll like it, I promise."

I wasn't sure what was going on but knew it was worth being patient to find out. After a five-block taxi ride, we pulled up in front of a charming neighborhood hotel I knew well. It was a European-boutique-style town house, and Gerald had booked a suite on the top floor. When we got settled in, I turned to him.

"Look, this is great as a treat, but what's the purpose? I've been patient, but it's driving me nuts. You've got to tell me now or I'll start screaming," I teased him.

Gerald just smiled and pointed to the corner of the room, where there was a large stone fireplace.

"I found the nicest hotel near us with a real wood-burning fireplace," he said. "How many times have you told me that you'd love to burn those things?" He glanced toward the suitcase stuffed with tampons. "Let's order a fabulous meal in the room and then have a bonfire."

I couldn't stop laughing. I'm sure a lot of paper products are used to start fires, but I don't know if a several-foot stack of tampons has ever served that purpose. It was the perfect way to celebrate my most visible marker of menopause. On that night, with a wonderful fire roaring in the background, even my dormant sexual desire made a brief return.

NINE

Bone and Body Boosters

BECAUSE I rarely eat dairy products, one of the menopausal conditions about which I was most concerned was the possible deterioration of my bones. It's frightening, but most of the bone loss in menopause happens at the very beginning, when estrogen and progesterone levels drop precipitously. We need to do something about this immediately. Starting a program a few years after entering menopause may be too late to avoid complications like osteoporosis. And osteoporosis is an insidious disease because you usually don't know you have it until you fracture a bone, or your posture is shot since your spine has curved so much.

Most of the recommendations to fight bone loss—primarily hormone replacement therapy—were already off my list. I learned that synthetic hormones do slow the rate of bone loss in menopausal women, and may sometimes even stop the loss, but they have to be used for many years—maybe for life—to have any effect. My first thought was that that result did not seem so difficult to duplicate naturally. Then I chanced upon a study that showed maybe I was setting my goal too low; research indicated that while estrogen replacement may halt bone loss, menopausal women who instead took calcium supplements and made lifestyle and dietary changes actually *gained* 11 percent bone mass in the first year, and more than half of them moved out of the so-called fracture zone. Since my bone density test had been sparkling only a few months earlier, I had a baseline by which I could eventually determine if my own program was working.

One highly touted drug for maintaining bone density is Fosamax, introduced in 1994. Since it is not a hormone and has been widely written about, it was the first thing I considered. Studies show that the drug can often increase bone mass. But Fosamax gives new meaning to the notion of side effects. It is extremely hard on the digestive tract. Patients on the drug are warned not to lie down for at least half an hour after taking it, lest they do serious damage to the esophagus. A New York friend of mine tried Fosamax, and her stomach was in turmoil after a couple of weeks, so she stopped. My mother-in-law in San Francisco tried it despite a long history of stomach ulcers. She lasted almost three weeks before having to abandon it because of burning sensations that doubled her over. I've had bouts with irritable bowel syndrome, so Fosamax sounded like something that might kick off a bad round of digestive ailments. Moreover, I found out that Fosamax itself is a synthetic product that doesn't exist anywhere in nature. And the bone it makes is a more brittle substance than human bone and may be more prone to fracture. On top of all this, doctors prescribing Fosamax think it probably requires a lifelong commitment; stopping could cause any bone gain to be lost immediately. Fosamax clearly was not going to become part of my natural approach to menopause.

Instead, I looked for ways to complement what I already did for maintaining healthy bones. For several years I had taken calcium supplements, between 500 and 750 milligrams a day. Without dairy in my diet, it was especially important that I take these supplements. And since vitamin D is essential to calcium absorption, I had either purchased calcium pills that were bundled with vitamin D or taken D separately. Magnesium was another mineral that I made part of my daily regimen, as it also helps with calcium absorption.

Now that I had read a bit more about calcium, I realized that as I entered menopause I needed more. So I upped my daily calcium intake to 1200 milligrams, and I split it so that half was taken in the morning and half in the evening. But I also discovered that if someone gets too much calcium, without the right balance of other minerals to help absorb it and metabolize it into an effective bone density booster, not only will it fail to work, but it might cause problems such as kidney stones. Too much of a good thing can do damage, and calcium is no different from many other vitamins and minerals. Many women just pop up to 1500 milligrams a day of calcium pills and assume they are helping their bones. Not necessarily. Balance is everything

in nature. It is the proper ratio of minerals, in conjunction
with one another, that determines whether your calcium
supplements are really helping your bones.

When I upped my dosage, I also switched to a liquid calcium in pill form, an easier way for the supplement to get
quickly absorbed into the body. There are a lot of calciums
on the market, and most of the cheaper ones are calcium
carbonate, otherwise known as chalk. Literally. It is mined
in the ground—not from any animal or plant source—and
is not always well absorbed. While calcium carbonate is
better than no supplement at all, if you can, opt for calcium
citrate, a form that is readily utilized by the body, especially in women over forty, who tend to have reduced stomach acid, which is required to absorb some of the other
brands. I also discovered that in addition to vitamin D and
magnesium, I needed vitamin K for bone mineralization,
and a minute amount, 3 milligrams, of the trace element
boron, which studies have shown is critical for optimal calcium metabolism.

Getting enough calcium is basic. But I knew I also had
to make more fundamental changes in both exercise and
diet. What it boiled down to was that I realized any bad
habits, like a poor diet or lack of exercise, that we could
have gotten away with when younger—combined with the
generally high level of stress in most of our lives, which
throws our hormonal systems completely out of whack—
make menopause much more difficult than it needs to be.

Further, I was convinced from my reading that diet may
play a bigger role in women's postmenopausal health than
even the levels of our hormones. For instance, doctors in the

United States pinpoint a lack of estrogen as one of the reasons women develop so many heart problems after menopause, and they like to cite studies that show hormone replacement helps protect the cardiovascular system. But contrast that with Thailand, where few menopausal women take hormones. There, only 7 percent of women die from heart problems, yet 63 percent of American women over the age of sixty-five die from heart ailments. The same is true of osteoporosis. The United States has one of the highest hip fracture rates in the world. Again, American doctors like to cite this as an inevitable curse of menopause and suggest that hormone replacement will keep bones strong. But women in a host of places, from Singapore to South Africa, have very low rates of hip fractures, sometimes only a twentieth of the U.S. figure. Why are their bones stronger, when in most of these places the women are not on hormone replacement therapy?

Even for breast cancer, countries like Taiwan and Japan have rates six times lower for women aged fifty and twenty times lower for postmenopausal women. If hormone loss is solely to blame for all these physical problems, why don't women in other parts of the globe experience them to the same extent as American women? I'm convinced that diet and lifestyle are major factors, and that the key is finding ways to naturally encourage the body to balance and heal itself. For me, this belief meant it wasn't too late to adopt a healthy program for both eating and exercising.

One important factor I had going for me was that I had given up my near pack-a-day smoking habit in my early thirties. Smoking isn't only a killer in terms of a host of cancers and heart disease; for women it is especially damaging. At menopause it can greatly exacerbate every bad symptom while slowing up all the good work you do to get your body and soul on track. Just on the question of bones, women who smoke have about a quarter less bone mass than those who don't smoke. Even going on hormone replacement therapy won't help, because smoking cancels out the benefits. So I figured I was ahead of where I would have been if I hadn't had the willpower to give up smoking.

Also, I'd been a regular exerciser for nearly a decade. I knew about its general benefits, but I didn't know until I did a little more reading that exercise helps normalize the hormones that are still produced by our bodies at menopause. That means it might help reduce cramping and minimize hot flashes. Exercise also helps the adrenal glands produce the estrogen we get after menopause. If you don't exercise, and you don't think you have the time for it because you are too busy with your job, family, and just getting through the average week, you're wrong. You can get going with only five minutes a day of some activity that raises your heart rate so you mildly perspire. Build that up to the point where you can work out several times a week, and you'll be doing yourself a big favor, especially during menopause. Dr. Susan Love, a prominent breast surgeon and women's health advocate, has said, "If there were a drug that had as many good effects as exercise has, we'd all be buying stock in it and getting rich."

I had not started exercising until I was in my midthirties. But even though working out next to all those twenty-something kids with near perfect bodies was pretty depressing in the beginning, I was soon convinced of the benefits of regular exercise and tried to get to the gym at least three times a week. I used a stationary bike or tread-mill for thirty to forty-five minutes, and often then took group classes for everything from ballet stretch and strengthening exercises to Pilates, a program of body align-ment and conditioning. But what I had never done was work out with weights, something Gerald did regularly. Now I began reading numerous articles and books that suggested that *only* weight-bearing and resistance exercises could put the demand on your body to strengthen your bones. Some studies showed that after forty-five years of age, which I had passed, even women who do active aerobic exercises rapidly lose lean muscle tissue and strength when passing through menopause. Other studies showed that using weights is the only way actually to *reverse* the loss of lean body tissue as well as bone density. I was obviously concerned about my bones, but I was also worried about that middle-aged spread around the midriff and thighs. Of course, my immediate worry was that if I began lifting weights I would bulk up with muscles and look too mascu-line. When I expressed that concern to a trainer at our gym, he laughed.

"That's the first thing I hear from almost every woman who starts working with weights," he said. "And if you think about it for a moment, you'll realize how silly it re-ally is. Look around at the men lifting heavy weights."

There were at least a dozen men working hard with free weights. "Do any of them look like Arnold Schwarzeneg-ger?" the trainer asked. Certainly not. A few were in good shape, but none of them looked remotely like a body-builder. "What about Gerald?" he asked. It was true that my own husband had worked hard with weights for six or seven years, and while he was very slim and muscular, he had certainly not bulked up.

"All these fellows you see in this gym," the trainer continued, "wish it would be so easy as to just pick up a weight and a few days later be bigger and more muscular. It just doesn't happen that way. It takes a lot of hard and regular work to build muscle, and men do it more easily anyway since they have natural growth hormone. You'll only be at risk if you start lifting very heavy weights, spend half a day at the gym, and eat and drink a lot of extra protein drinks to add mass. If you start lifting weights and do the right type of weight-bearing exercise, all that is going to happen is that you'll build up some strength." And help my bones, I thought to myself.

I decided that I would use Gerald as my trainer. If my own husband didn't have the patience to give me a good exercise regime, then who could? The first day he tried to show me how to use a curved bar with two five-pound plates at each end to do a bicep exercise. I was so weak that I dropped it after two repetitions, missing his foot by a fraction of an inch. Breaking his foot would have been one way to ensure that my husband passed me along to a personal trainer. But luckily, since it missed, he stayed with me. Although he worked with me on a tough five-day-a-week schedule in the beginning, I did notice that he tended to stand a little farther away after that near miss.

Two days a week I would work on those body parts

that require pulling motions for each exercise—the back and biceps. Two other days were set aside for so-called push exercises, involving the chest, triceps, and shoulders. Wednesdays were reserved for leg exercises, in which I used the machines at the gym to try to make my thighs and bum firm and perky. And I was pleasantly surprised to learn that none of my workouts required heavy weights—I quickly discovered that my muscles would get quite shocked just from lifting the tiniest weights at the club. After each weight workout I would still do half an hour on a treadmill or stepping machine to keep my cardiovascular system in tiptop shape. On weekends, my two days off, you couldn't pay me to go near a gym. I had never worked as hard at fitness, and I really looked forward to my off time. Especially since I was spending more time at the gym, I was now getting up an hour earlier each morning so I wouldn't cut into my real workday. I also knew that while I was sticking to an arduous schedule to see what, if any, difference it would make now that I was in menopause, the good news was that, once I reached any goals, maintaining the benefits would take just a few hours a week.

Within a few months I observed noticeable changes from the weight-bearing work. I felt stronger, leaner, and fitter than I had in years. All the classes I had taken during the past decade hadn't made the difference that weights wrought in a short time. And instead of looking bigger or too muscular, I now had good tone in my arms, legs, and chest. For instance, among many visible changes, that horrible flap of skin under the arms that seems so loose as we get older, no matter how thin we are, had suddenly firmed.

My shoulders seemed straighter, my overall posture better, and there was slight definition on parts of my body where I never knew I had muscles. I was also definitely more flexible.

"Whoa, what have you been doing?" a high-pitched voice said behind me one day at the gym. I wasn't sure the question was directed at me, but I turned around. There was a woman I knew only casually. Dubbed Dragon Mouth by most of us who knew her, she had a wicked tongue and never kept her opinions to herself. She always seemed critical of someone or something.

"What do you mean?" I asked, half expecting her to accuse me of having left some perspiration on the bike I'd used or forgetting to put away an exercise mat from the last class.

"Well, look at you," she said, staring at me from my head to my toes. "You certainly have done something different. You look so toned; it looks great on you. Whatever you're doing, keep it up, dear."

I sighed with relief. "Thank you."

An actual compliment from Dragon Mouth. That was the best confirmation to date that my new exercise routine was really working.

TEN

Eating My Way Through Menopause

ONE of the biggest surprises I noticed after starting my weight regimen was that, after a couple of months of working with weights, I thought some of my trousers seemed looser around the waist and hips. Not sure if it was real or just wishful thinking, I decided to step on a scale, something I rarely did. I was quite astonished to see that my weight had dropped by nearly five pounds, precisely the opposite of what I had been told was supposed to be happening during menopause.

It turns out that strength training revs up your metabolism, so you burn more calories no matter what you're doing, even sitting in front of your computer. That helps, since a woman's metabolism slows about 2 percent a year starting in middle age. Also, pound for pound, muscle burns more calories than fat. Because I had added muscle, I was automatically burning more calories each day, helping me keep trimmer than ever.

Of course, these results did not come about because I went to the gym for an hour a day and then spent the rest of the time stuffing my face full of potato chips, fried chicken, hamburgers and fries, and wedges of chocolate cake. I was always a large eater. "There's a three-hundred-pound woman waiting to burst out of there one day," Gerald used to tease me. Once, at a dinner party, someone asked Gerald's editor Bob Loomis whether I had a good appetite. "Oh, Trisha eats like a bird," Bob said. "A vulture." But I countered the quantities by sticking to relatively healthy food. For years I had avoided anything deep-fried; broiling, baking, poaching, steaming, sautéing, and stir-frying left me plenty of tasty ways to prepare food without the heavy fats and high calories. I had also gradually cut down on butter, cheese, and rich desserts. Red meat was not something I liked, but I ate a lot of chicken, fish, and vegetables, almost always grilled. (If you like red meat, it's probably wise to cut back on your portions, since it is high in saturated fat, low in nutrients, has few antioxidants and no fiber, and is calorie dense.) As for other meats, such as chicken, if it had the skin still on when served in a restaurant, I would eat everything but that fatty layer.

So over time this way of eating became a lifestyle, not a diet. Before I started my new routine, my weight varied little, usually ranging between 127 and 132 pounds on my five-foot-seven frame. Yet I knew from the test a few months earlier that my body fat was higher than I wanted.

So, with this new exercise routine, I thought it also prudent to modify my diet.

At menopause, I learned, it becomes more important than ever to find a way of eating that complements the changes under way instead of fighting them. Menopause is often associated with a more matronly body, and that pre-conception has some basis in the physiological changes we undergo. It's not only that we add weight—about ten pounds for the average woman over a two- to three-year span—but also what bothers most women is a redistribution of existing fat. Estrogen, which rounds out our bodies at puberty, has the opposite effect when it falls off. As fat declines in the round parts—the hips, butt, and breasts—it moves to the stomach and sometimes upper body. We get that wonderfully thick look that screams, "Middle age!"

If you really want to counter this and at least keep the same body you had in your thirties, it's certainly not enough to follow the typical advice of eating more fruits and vegetables and cutting back on saturated fat (although none of that is bad advice, especially given a Harvard study a few years back that found that women who ate the most fruit and vegetables had about a 40 percent lower risk of developing breast cancer than those who ate the least). Getting our diets in balance as we pass through menopause takes into account a lot of things happening to our bodies beyond just calories.

For instance, maintaining a steady blood sugar level can make a significant difference in how you feel emotionally and physically during menopause. Steady blood sugar helps your body fully utilize whatever hormones you still have and helps protect against some of the wild fluctuations to which the body can otherwise be prone. Every time we eat refined carbohydrates like sugars, white flours, most breads and cereals, cakes, candy, cookies, and the like, we set off an insulin reaction in our bodies. Our energy is boosted for a short while after the insulin is released, but when it returns to normal or drops even lower, we feel sluggish. And worse, we feel hungry for the same foods that set off the reaction in the first place. This is part of a vicious cycle that can eventually lead to diabetes in some people and in others a form of glucose intolerance. For the latter group, eating simple carbohydrates, even in light amounts, can lead to weight gain and puffiness.

Some culprits, I thought, such as sugar itself, too much salt, and excessive caffeine, would be easy to restrict. Sugar has no nutrient value but calories, and whatever the body doesn't use as energy it just converts to fat. I certainly didn't need that at any time, much less in menopause, with my metabolism naturally slowing down. Moreover, high sugar intake can actually limit one's ability to absorb calcium and in some cases can deplete it from the body, just the opposite of what I needed for my bones. Some studies even show that sugar can exacerbate hot flashes, water retention, and bloating and cramping. As for salt, excessive amounts not only can lead to high blood pressure but can aggravate menopausal symptoms, including bloating, breast tenderness, and headaches. It also can cause calcium to be excreted instead of absorbed into our bones.

The problem, I soon discovered, was that while I might

not add sugar or salt to the things I ate, both were hidden ingredients in some of my favorite prepared and processed foods. Reading the labels carefully made a big difference. For instance, among several high-fiber cereals from which I could choose, only one—Fiber One—had no sugar, whereas the others had between 7 and 11 grams per serving. Since they all tasted much the same and offered nearly identical nutritional benefits and high fiber, I opted for the one with no added sugar. I was able to make similar substitutions for a whole range of prepared foods. One example, which might seem unlikely, is seafood cocktail sauce. It was something I'd regularly buy in the supermarket to use when I got some fresh shrimp or crabs at the local fishmonger. One brand from my local market had been my steady choice until I noticed that its 10-ounce jar held 3200 milligrams of sodium, a day and a half's total supply. I did a little label reading and soon found another brand—Trader Joe's—that tasted just as good and had, in an 11-ounce jar, only 620 milligrams of sodium, a fifth of my regular one. And some of my favorite processed foods had "hidden" sodium in the form of flavor enhancers and preservatives such as MSG. It did not take long to realize that being label savvy would help me cut back on some of the ingredients that were no longer my friends.

Caffeine was a bit easier to regulate. I was surprised to learn that just 300 milligrams—the amount in two mugs of coffee—is enough to raise your blood pressure and push your kidneys into overdrive, thereby depleting key vitamins and minerals like C, the B complex, calcium, magnesium, and zinc. The amount of caffeine in three cups of coffee drains about 45 milligrams of calcium from your bones. My saving grace on caffeine is that I never really overloaded on it. Although I was raised in England, I never developed a liking for tea, another potent source of caffeine. And I grew up without soft drinks and therefore never acquired a taste for them. Studies show that the average American actually drinks more soft drinks than water each day. If you're a soft drink fan, do yourself a favor and at least switch to brands that are decaffeinated. Even then, proceed with caution, because all soft drinks contain a lot of extra phosphorus—if you have too much phosphorus, calcium will be lost from your body every time you go to the bathroom.

On the Internet one night I came across some recent studies that surprised me about the poor condition most American women are in in terms of weight. Over half in their fifties are overweight, the highest percentage of any age-group. I was aware of the risks of being heavy, from high blood pressure and hardening of the arteries to diabetes. If I ever had any doubt that some extra pounds could make a difference, a recent study involving 115,000 women revealed that the leanest women, including those 15 to 20 percent below the average weight, had the lowest death rates. Even middle-aged women of average weight had a 30 percent greater risk of dying than those who weighed less. That study, the largest of its kind, corrected for women who were smokers or had preexisting conditions like cancer, heart disease, or diabetes. It concluded that "being overweight is second only to cigarette smoking as a cause of premature death."

Staying healthy was enough of an incentive for me to try to stay lean, but it also had a lot to do with my positive self-image, and not wanting to upset my mental or emotional balance through menopause. I don't aspire to mimic the waiflike models in fashion magazines who appear to be in desperate need of a good meal, but I do like being trim and fit. If suddenly I found my body spreading out beyond my control, it was not going to make me feel as though the move into this new phase of life was all positive and empowering. I had tackled changes in exercise and diet not only for the important benefits inside my body, like those to my bones, but also to reap the benefits on the outside, the all-important psychological shell of how we look and how that often affects how we feel about ourselves. This may or may not be important to you, but it was to me.

Although I thought I ate very healthily, I decided it was time to really test what regularly passed through my mouth and went straight to my hips. As with many aspects of figuring out the right mix for menopause, it took a little extra work. For a week I marked down everything I ate, then logged on to the Internet and calculated the carbohydrates, fat, and protein in my typical weekly diet. To my surprise, I was overloaded on carbohydrates—breads, rice, pasta—and underweighted in protein—lean meat and fish. Only 20 percent of my diet was fat, but 65 percent was carbohydrates, and about 15 percent was protein. I decided to reduce sharply the carbohydrates, especially sugar and many processed foods, and instead rely more on high-fiber and vitamin-rich complex carbs like grains, beans, and vegetables, as well as boost my protein intake. My new guidelines were also to emphasize whole, fresh foods, limiting the packaged goods I bought.

Out was my daily large bagel, which I was surprised to learn supplied an entire day's quota of carbohydrates in a single serving. Also gone were the bowls of pasta at Italian restaurants and the cartons of fried rice from my nearby Chinese take-out. At restaurants, where I used to start devouring the bread when it was put on the table, I now steered clear unless the bread was very special. Meanwhile, salmon, red snapper, or sea bass replaced the pasta dinners, and fried rice gave way to grilled chicken breasts and assorted greens. My bagel became a bowl of fresh fruit.

I picked foods that I knew I could live with. This could not be a diet; it had to be a way of life. That meant I wasn't ready to give up everything I liked, or else there was no chance I could stick with it for the long term. I also needed a way of eating that fit my lifestyle, which meant eating out often at restaurants and frequent traveling. My new foods had to be things I could easily order off a menu as well as prepare at home.

So I stayed with coffee, although I cut back on the amount of caffeine by mixing half decaffeinated with full caffeine in the morning and afternoon, then switching to full decaf by the evening. I enjoy a glass of wine several times a week, so that stayed in my routine despite the books that counsel against alcohol. (Most of the literature indicates that menopausal women who have more than two drinks a day have higher production of estrogens tied to breast cancer development, plus a worsening of some symptoms. Unfortunately, we simply don't metabolize alcohol as well as men. On the plus side, although I don't like the taste of beer, bourbon, gin, or whiskey, they all have differing amounts of plant estrogens, which may help counter some of menopause's symptoms.)

It was easy to stay away from food I dislike, such as red meat, dairy products, or a lot of salt, but I must admit I did miss my extra piles of warm bread and an occasional plate of French fries for quite a few months. When I was a kid I used to slather so much butter on my bread that it was often the subject du jour for our family, especially since I was so skinny; no one could understand why I wasn't a butterball. But I had slowly cut back on eating butter, and it was not hard now to keep it out of my diet. The same was true for cheese; it became an ingredient to sprinkle on top of salads and other dishes, as opposed to a chunk that would have passed as a snack a year earlier.

There were also some foods I had never particularly liked, such as tofu. Girls, I know many of you just wrinkled your noses and shook your heads no. I did the same thing, but once I learned how helpful it is during menopause, I decided it was worthwhile to find some way to mix tofu into my daily routine. I'm pretty open to change, so I figured the worst thing that could happen was I wouldn't like the new recipes. Not a big risk. And actually I found a lot of interesting ways to use tofu—barbecuing it, grilling slices with some chopped peanuts on top, or sautéing it into an omelet. It's worth the effort, since tofu has high concentrations of soy, which contains a couple of compounds—phytoestrogens—that have a mild hormonal effect. Soy is a virtual wonder food. It offers help to your heart by lowering cholesterol, aids your bones by increasing calcium absorption, and, as opposed to estrogen, it can actually *lower* your risk of several cancers. Other good sources of phytoestrogens include cashews, peanuts, almonds, flaxseed, celery, parsley, figs, dates, and apricots. These foods—including some packaged products found in your local supermarket, like soy burgers—can give you the benefits that estrogen might provide in minimizing menopausal problems without any of the downside, such as stimulation of estrogen receptors in the breasts that increase cancer risk. Once, at my local supermarket, I had just put a couple of boxes of soy burgers in my basket when a real Romeo type, who had been following at some safe distance, decided this gave him an opening for a conversation.

"Hey, veggie burgers. Are you a vegetarian?"

I was late for an appointment and not in the mood for idle chitchat. I swung around and looked at him very firmly. Somehow, the first thing that popped into my head came out of my mouth: "It's all about estrogen receptors, Bubba."

Quite bewildered, he left me alone.

Although you, too, may have to run the gauntlet of bad pickup lines at your local market, keep an eye out for products packed with soy. And although I also use soy supplements, I try to get as much soy as possible from food.

Soon, I had a new typical day's menu. Breakfast consists of several mixed high-fiber cereals, low in sugar. Sometimes I add a few pieces of fruit. Most mornings I grind a tablespoon of flaxseed and sprinkle it on the cereal. Flaxseed has precursors that your body turns into very weak estrogens.

The coffee is my half-decaf/half-caf blend. Mid-morning, after my workout, I have some fruit, often a banana and mango, and some fresh juice. Lunch varies but is often a large bowl of soup that has no dairy, a mixed-green salad tossed with some grilled slices of tofu and a very light vinaigrette dressing, and a plate of lean cold cuts or a chicken breast. I'll usually have more coffee at lunch, but sometimes I switch to spring water. I drink at least eight large glasses of water a day, so lunch is a good time to start. I know many women think of drinking water as a nutritional penance of sorts, but it's pretty easy once you get used to it. (If you need help, just add a dash of citrus juice.) Those of you who want to get your liquids in tea should be aware that if you drink it with meals, tea's natural tannin binds to important minerals like calcium and keeps them from being digested.

During the afternoon, my regular snack is a local frozen yogurt treat called Tasti-D-Lite; although it is filled with sugar and counters my guidelines, it fits with my overall view that you can't deprive yourself of everything you like but just have to do it in moderation. And it is also the best evidence that many of the things we eat as comfort food, or as guilty-pleasure snacks, have tasty and healthier versions available if we look around a little.

Dinner, against the advice of most nutritionists, is usually my largest meal, often consisting of a large tossed salad with bits of barbecued tofu and a main dish of grilled fish or chicken, some lightly grilled vegetables, and occasionally a small side of lentils or couscous. Some nights I have a platter of sushi, one of my favorites. Once in a while it's veggie burgers or soy hot dogs. Other times it might be cold poached salmon. Often I have a glass of white wine. Dessert is invariably fresh fruit. And at night, between more water or juice, I usually end with a final sweet, either a low-fat pudding or a chocolate GeniSoy protein bar, a delicious, fat-free treat packed with vitamins and soy.

After a month of adjustments, I took notes on another week of eating. This time the fat was still about 20 percent, but protein was now more than 30 percent of my diet, and carbohydrates were less than half. I could see the difference in my clothes. Things fit a little looser. A couple of bumps on the sides of my thighs had, at long last, mercifully disappeared. And my waist seemed narrower. After two more months I finally had the courage to step on a scale again. Another 6 pounds less, just under 120, a weight I hadn't seen in many years. And considering that I had been putting on muscle through my workouts, I was ecstatic. After three months I had my body fat retested. It had dropped to 26 percent from its original 34. Over the next six months it would drop as low as 15 percent, more than half of where I started.

As the months passed, I not only grew to really like my new and nutritious way of eating but also found that, when I did veer too far off my regimen, I didn't feel as good. I am more sluggish if I eat a lot of fats than if I keep my food clean. Once, at a dinner party, the only dish served was beef swimming in a rich béarnaise sauce. Although I ate only a little bit, I felt like it sat in my stomach all night. Gerald, eventually growing tired of my groaning, presented me with a platter of Tums once we got home.

When a restaurant offers a dish saturated in butter, or too thick a cream sauce, instead of ordering it that way and later feeling heavy, almost queasy, I ask for it simply grilled, with the sauce served on the side. I know some of my friends are afraid to speak up when they dine out, somehow feeling that special requests are a burden on the kitchen. But my view is that you are paying for it, and it is your body, so don't be afraid to ask for the dish to be prepared the way you want. Most restaurants, in this day and age of increased health consciousness, are quite willing to accommodate simple requests.

This entire changeover was made easier because Gerald decided to join me in my healthier way of eating. I knew from my research that what I had devised was not merely a women's diet, but I wasn't sure if Gerald wanted to go along. Once he did, though, it made my sticking to it much less difficult.

A few months after I'd started on my regime, Gerald and I visited some friends at the beach in New Jersey. During the day we wandered along the boardwalk, and my girlfriend bought a container of thick-cut French fries. I passed and ordered a lemonade. She knew that I used to be a big fan of fries and was surprised I wasn't having any.

"It's simple," I told her. "I like fries. But I like the way I look now even more."

As far as my physique was concerned, I did not have the normal effects of menopause. There was no thickening middle, no extra rolls of fat, and no loss of lean muscle tissue. In fact, between the weight-bearing exercises and the

carbohydrate-reduced diet, I not only maintained where I was when I began menopause but dramatically improved. And I certainly seemed to have more energy; some menopausal women experience a sharp drop-off of energy because of reduced testosterone levels. The changes I had witnessed certainly confirmed that it is never too late to start eating right.

As for the effect of all this exercise and good food on my bones, that would have to wait for another bone density test. I had decided to put a year between the exams. I could only hope that the internal results were as good as the changes I was witnessing on the outside.

ELEVEN

Only Skin Deep

WHILE I was working on keeping my body in shape, I figured there was no sense in letting my face and hair go to pot. In a cruel trick of nature, as if it's not bad enough that menopause can induce such unpleasantries as hot flashes, it also tends to dry the skin and affect the hair. No wonder so many menopausal woman feel blue at some point—you're going through all of these biological and mental challenges at the same time that simple things like hair and skin appear to be going through the reverse of puberty.

I have naturally curly hair. When I was a teenager I generally hated it and had it straightened. But after most of my hair broke off, I decided I'd get used to it curly. There were days I had to battle the frizzes and other times I had to weather periods when fashion mavens in New York declared curly hair "out," but on the whole I had come to rather like it.

Now, all of a sudden, I noticed that my hair seemed much drier, the texture was coarser, and it was not as manageable. Initially I thought it might be my imagination, from having read too many books about the possible side effects of menopause. But I was soon disabused of that notion on one visit to my hairdresser.

"What have you been doing to your hair?" he asked.

"What do you mean?"

"Well, maybe the question is what *haven't* you been doing to your hair? I've never seen it in such poor condition."

I am meticulous about my hair. I get it trimmed every six weeks, condition it daily, and use a host of products intended to enhance the shine and texture. This news did not make me happy.

He didn't have to say anything about my skin. I had noticed that I was getting dry patches around the chin and on my cheeks. I had never had that in my life. Never even had pimples as a teenager. My skin has that milky-white English tone, and I've always received compliments on it. I haven't sunbathed in fifteen years, and I slather myself with sunblock when venturing outside. I gave up smoking at the same time I stopped being a sun worshiper. Now I was confronting my first skin problems in years. I knew from my early research that lowered hormones played a role. As hormone levels drop, our skin gets drier and thinner and cannot produce as much oil. This is combined with other effects of aging, in which the skin loses fat under its top layers—making for that wonderful look where the skin is loose, sags here and there, and the wrinkles stand out more prominently. To make matters worse, by the time we reach menopause, much of the damage to our skin has already been done from years of things like sun, smoking, other environmental abuse, stress, yo-yo dieting, you name it. Just what I needed on top of hot flashes.

When I tried to cover the dry patches with makeup, it invariably made my skin look even drier. Although there is little scientific proof that hormone replacement makes the skin look younger or smoother, the articles I had read were replete with horror stories about women who refused to take hormones, so their skin looked like leather. And while I was realistic enough to know I was not going to have young skin again, I did want to make sure my skin was healthy, radiating vitality in both tone and texture.

The afternoon I left the beauty salon, I was off to the library. It was time to do some research on whether there might be remedies for my skin and hair. I chanced across a supplement my mother had spoken about years earlier—evening primrose oil. It contains an essential fatty acid that we need for both skin and hair. Few of us get enough of it through food, since its major sources are walnuts and pumpkin seeds (off my list as too high in calories and fat) and oily fish like mackerel, sardines, and wild trout (fish I just seem never to eat). Also, the foods give us only a simplified version of the proper fatty acid. Since many of our bodies are so corroded by a typical Western diet too high in fat, we have difficulty converting that simple fatty acid in the foods into the one we really need. And as we get older the enzymes in our bodies that help this conversion break down. All these hurdles are overcome with a single daily dose of evening primrose oil (besides helping hair and skin, some studies show that evening primrose oil helps alleviate PMS symptoms and may actually reduce benign breast cysts. I began taking 1000 milligrams a day, split between two capsules, one in the morning with breakfast and one in the evening with dinner. And vitamin C, which was part of my regular daily supplements, promotes collagen production, which helps the skin seem more elastic. Collagen is one of the key substances we have less of as estrogen drops.

I discovered that a handful of herbs—including burdock root, red clover, and echinacea—are successful in combating dry skin, even in more severe cases, like full-blown eczema. That afternoon I stopped by a local health shop and bought some capsules of those herbs. The clerk there also recommended two other supplements, both of which I later checked on at the library. Selenium, a trace element, was part of my routine as a general immune system booster, and I now learned that it is also important in maintaining the elasticity of skin. And 25 milligrams a day of silica, a form of the mineral silicon, is also a good idea to enhance the skin's appearance.

At the same time I added these supplements, I decided to change the facial moisturizer creams I had been using. I have sensitive skin, so a lot of moisturizers don't work for me. I was looking for a richer cream that would really nourish and pamper my skin without causing any irritation. Although some articles on natural remedies recommended a cream made of licorice and German chamomile, that was really intended more to treat the dry patches than to moisturize the skin. I wanted a normal moisturizer that would complement my new herbal and mineral supplements.

Over a couple of weeks I tried several highly touted moisturizers made by Kiehl's, Clinique, and Prescriptives. None completely worked. At Bloomingdale's one day, frustrated that I had not yet settled on the right moisturizer, I wandered around the cosmetic counters, studying samples and talking to some of the saleswomen. One young woman, who seemed particularly helpful, leaned across the counter after a few minutes of conversation, and whispered, "I really shouldn't be telling you this, since I should sell you something we make." She looked over her shoulder to make sure that none of her co-workers was listening. Since this was Manhattan and Bloomingdale's, I half expected her to suggest some exotic concoction that I would have to import from Rangoon or some other inaccessible corner of the globe.

"Go to Avon," she said. "They have the best new products. I use them myself."

Her skin was remarkable, but that was the last brand name I expected. "Avon calling" was a joke among many of my friends, who viewed the company as a quaint throwback to Ozzie and Harriet days. I had been an Avon girl as a teenager, and although I am pretty good at sales, it was the one job at which I actually lost money. She sensed that I was skeptical.

"It's not your mother's Avon," she assured me. "Give them a try."

"But I don't want to have one of those salesladies coming by my apartment with a suitcase of samples."

"It's the nineties." She smiled. "I order mine from their Web site."

An Internet site was a good omen that Avon might have truly updated itself. That evening I logged on to Avon.com and soon ordered several products that sounded promising, all from the Anew and Hydrofirming lines. It did not take me long to become a complete convert. I am convinced that the Avon creams—which are hypoallergenic and won't clog pores or cause blemishes—have hydrated my skin like no other cream I've ever used.

I have a regular routine: I clean my face with only water in the morning, then use a daytime moisturizer that has a sun protection factor of 15. Over that I put on my makeup. At night I use a nonsoap cleanser—my favorite is Cetaphil—because almost anything else, including toners, is just too drying and astringent at this time in your life. Then I use a Hydrofirming overnight moisturizer and a Hydrofirming eye gel that has a slightly lighter consistency than the face cream.

In a couple of weeks I saw noticeable results in both the resiliency and the firmness of my skin. Within a month I was once again getting compliments on my skin, something that had stopped when I began menopause. I knew the Avon products must have been working when Gerald not only asked me questions about them but also started using some himself.

The richness of the Avon creams may have helped, but I still believe that the herbal supplements got rid of my dry patches. It also didn't hurt that I was drinking at least eight glasses of water daily, enough to keep my skin well hydrated. I took the herbs for nearly three months to ensure that the patches were history, then continued using the Avon creams and the evening primrose oil capsules on their own. During the winter months, when apartments in New York tend to be very drying because of overheating, I run a small humidifier in the bedroom overnight. That is still my regimen, and after two years my skin looks better than when I entered menopause.

As for my hair, I believe that my general regimen for skin actually helped it, too. One of the problems with hair and menopause is that the hair seems thinner because the skin around the follicles tends to lose collagen and therefore its support. There is also reduced blood flow to the scalp, providing less nourishment to the hair. The things I was doing to enhance my skin obviously offered benefits to my scalp. Evening primrose oil is often recommended on its own for helping people with thinning hair. But I added a few other tricks. Whenever I washed my hair I used warm water, then rinsed it out with cool water to increase circulation to the scalp. I stayed away from any shampoos or hairstyling products that had drying alcohol. And I switched to new products that promised more moisturizers and fewer chemicals in my daily washing and conditioning. After a trial-and-error approach, I settled on a product line from Aveda, sold in their own stores as well as in cosmetic and drugstores. I noticed a difference in the shine and texture of my hair after using those products for only a few weeks, and again, I have stayed with them ever since.

. . .

Obviously, changes in hair and skin are two of the symptoms that seem least important during menopause, especially compared with strong bones and a healthy heart. But
such external things can affect how you feel about yourself.
They may be only the superficial bad effects of this midlife
change, but countering them provides an easy-to-see confirmation that your natural program is working.

TWELVE

The Vitamin and Herb Shop

RECENTLY I met a friend who was visiting from California. Gerald and I went to join her and her husband for an early breakfast at their midtown hotel. After we placed our orders, I took out a couple of small pillboxes and put them near my coffee cup.

"What are those?" my friend asked.

"Oh, just the vitamins and minerals I take every day."

She seemed flabbergasted. "I take a daily and some extra vitamin C, but I've never seen so many pills. What are they all for?"

"Each one has a little story. Are you sure you want to hear it?"

She nodded. Gerald, who knew the stories, began talking to her husband about the latest developments in computers, his default subject of interest if I get waylaid into a discussion about menopause or health.

Until my friend had pointed it out that morning, I had lost sight of how many supplements I had slowly added during menopause. During the course of a day—because I split some of the dosages into two portions—I take almost twenty pills. I know most of you girls just shook your head and said, "That's crazy, I couldn't do that." But then, I think it's probably crazy to go ahead and pop a single pill— hormone replacements—that might well accomplish less than my basket of supplements and runs the real, even if small, risk of inducing cancer. I'll gladly go through the extra effort of multiple supplements if doing so means I'll gain the equivalent of a free pass through menopause and be relieved of my fear of breast cancer.

The supplements I use were not the first ones I grabbed at the health food shop, but rather the survivors of a months-long process of trial and error. They were win-nowed from a large list by checking information both in the library and on the Internet. I not only looked for the benefits they could provide but carefully checked for possible side effects or bad interactions between them.

If you think that most supplements are unnecessary, that eating a balanced diet and a single multivitamin gives us all the nutrients we need, you need to rethink, as I did. My eyes opened when I chanced across a recent Department of Agriculture three-day survey of the food intake of 21,500 people. Not a *single* person consumed 100 percent of the recommended daily requirement of ten basic nutrients. Other government-sponsored studies reveal that half of the entire population has marginal nutritional deficiencies.

What I wanted in supplements were vitamins and herbs

that would actually strengthen my body and my immune system while providing some of the same protections promised by hormone replacement therapy, both in relieving my menopause symptoms and in giving protection to my heart and bones. But I never lost sight of the fact that nutritional supplements are just that—supplements, not substitutes for a good and healthy lifestyle.

I broke the supplements into two general groups. The first included basic nutrition with an emphasis on antioxidants. The second was focused specifically on menopause, alleviating symptoms while supercharging the body's strength.

When I started menopause, I already took a multivitamin, what I consider the basic starting point. A good multivitamin is also the first wall of defense against so-called free radicals, toxic molecules and atoms that can, if they get out of hand, destroy body tissue and cell walls, leading to arteriosclerosis, cancer, dementia, arthritis, and age-related problems ranging from wrinkled skin and poor eyesight to failing memory. Free radicals are inevitable, but they are more likely to proliferate if our bodies are subjected to a lot of stress, chemical or electromagnetic exposure, or heavy physical demands. Poor nutrition can also set them off. As you might imagine, menopause is one of those times when it is especially wise to be ensuring that free radicals don't get out of control. It is also a good time, because of the real stresses we are physically and mentally enduring, to ensure that our bodies are getting all the nutrient protection possible.

Centrum was my choice for a multi, but Theragran-M or

any equivalent generic is fine. I like Centrum because, as opposed to some multis, it also includes small amounts of some necessary minerals. Important ones are potassium, for muscles; selenium, which works synergistically with vitamin E and protects the immune system by destroying excessive free radicals; zinc, which is necessary not only for protein synthesis and healthy skin and bones but also for ridding the body of toxic pollutants; iron, which a lot of women are deficient in as we age; and molybdenum, a trace mineral that helps in the absorption of the iron.

Almost all multis provide 100 percent of the government's recommended daily allowance for major vitamin groups such as A, D, and E. I thought that was pretty good until I read that the government levels are really the very basic minimums. They are established only to prevent nutrition-deficiency diseases such as scurvy (a lack of vitamin C) and beriberi (too little vitamin B_1). Those government minimums are almost certainly not enough if you want additional nutritional benefits. Under physical stress from our polluted environment, and psychological stress from our high-octane lifestyles, nutrients are depleted from our bodies at rates unknown by our ancestors. In many cases, and particularly as our bodies pass menopause, we simply need certain vitamins and nutrients in larger quantities. For instance, the recommended daily allowance for vitamin E is 30 IU. Many of you who take supplements already take far more than that, in part because studies showing dosages more than ten times that have had a host of beneficial effects. I had had to double my daily E intake from 400 to 800 IU to alleviate my hot flashes. That's more than twenty-five times the government's recommended dosage. So you won't be surprised that some other vitamins also need a little boosting above what a normal multi provides.

When it comes to the antioxidants, it is particularly important to increase some of the dosages beyond those provided in the multi. After my research, I felt comfortable with adding the following amounts, which I dubbed power boosters.

· *An additional 25,000 IU of beta-carotene.* A precursor to vitamin A, beta-carotene is indispensable in fighting free radicals, protecting the immune system, guarding against premature aging, and fighting infection and even, in some studies, cancer. The liver converts beta-carotene into vitamin A as the body needs it. Although it is found in green, leafy vegetables, few of us get enough of it through food. The reason I add extra beta-carotene, and not vitamin A directly, is that vitamin A can build up in the body, and too much can be toxic. Beta-carotene does not store in the body, and when we have enough vitamin A, we simply won't convert any more of the beta-carotene we take.

· *An extra 100 micrograms of selenium.* A good multi, even if it includes selenium, will usually have only 20 milligrams. To get any real advantage from this important antioxidant, you need somewhere between 50 and 200 micrograms a day. You can get it from food, but unless you are eating a lot of Brazil nuts, brown rice, liver, molasses, wheat germ, or sea plants, you're likely not getting enough. I keep my total dosage of selenium in the middle of the recommended amount, since it is toxic at high levels—over 3000 micrograms a day—and can hurt the nervous system. Remember, one of the first things I learned about vitamins and minerals is that just because something is good for you, more of it isn't necessarily better. Keep your dosages sane.

· *An additional 800 IU of vitamin E.* This fights my hot flashes. When I believe that I am past the point of getting hot flashes, I will cut my vitamin E back to 400 IU. It's a great all-around antioxidant, and particularly during menopause it helps circulation, blood sugar problems, and even the formation of benign breast lumps. You can get a lot of E from nuts, seeds, brown rice, wheat germ, and dark green, leafy vegetables. But, again, if you are like me, you probably need the supplement. From what I read, this is one vitamin for which the body evidently can't recognize the difference between the synthetic and the natural. I've seen some studies that advocate up to 2000 IU a day for therapeutic purposes, but that seems awfully high to me. I would add what it takes to work—in my case, 800 IU. Keep in mind that if you have high blood pressure, megadoses of E might worsen your condition. Also, if you're going to have any surgery, stop taking vitamin E for a week or so beforehand—like aspirin, it can make you bleed a bit more. Finally, there are some preliminary and contradictory studies indicating that if you've had breast cancer, too much E may not be a good thing, so until more definitive data is available, you might be careful about upping the dose without first asking your doctor.

· *1000 milligrams extra of vitamin C.* Vitamin C is such an important antioxidant because of its key role in many parts of the immune system, including the formation of collagen and connective tissue in skin, cartilage, and tendons. This helps counteract the tendency for skin to dry out after menopause. Vitamin C also supports the adrenal glands in manufacturing basic hormones like adrenaline, and this is especially important in menopause since the adrenals take over this responsibility from the ovaries, which have shut down. Many nutritionists recommend between 1000 and 3000 milligrams a day. I get 60 milligrams in my multi and add 1000 milligrams in a pill later in the day. Vitamin C is water-soluble, so if you take too much, the body will just get rid of the excess. That's why I spend a few dollars more and make sure my C supplements are time-released, so that the 1000 milligrams don't just get passed out of my body but are released steadily through the day.

· *At least 15 milligrams of zinc.* Again, my multi gives me 15 milligrams, but I double that with an extra zinc supplement. The body gets the most protection if you get between 30 and 45 milligrams of zinc a day. You might be able to get by on just your multi if you eat a lot of liver, pecans, mushrooms, oysters, egg yolks, sunflower seeds, and the like. These aren't a steady or big part of my diet, so I make sure I get the 30 milligrams through supplements. At the health food store, look for either zinc citrate or zinc picolinate—they are the most easily absorbed.

· *Essential fatty acids.* Don't let the name scare you, girls. Essential fatty acids *don't* make you fat! Earlier, when describing what I did to protect my skin and hair, I mentioned evening primrose oil. It is basically an essential fatty acid called gamma-linolenic acid (GLA). This and several other essential fatty acids—including the omega family—are critical in boosting the immune system and are found in every cell of our bodies. These essential fatty acids have a positive effect on whatever hormone production we are left with after menopause, as well as helping the same areas that hormone replacement does, such as preventing heart disease, arteriosclerosis, and high blood pressure. Normally, our bodies just convert the fat we eat into the necessary essential fatty acids. However, if we are deficient in certain vitamins, take in too much junk food, or eat only a little fat, our bodies can have trouble converting the food to the right types of protective fatty acids. Deficiencies can lead to heart disease, cancer, arthritis, allergies, and several immune-related disorders. Since our bodies can't manufacture them, we have to get these acids from food or supplements. I am pretty strict about limiting the amount of fat in my diet, so I do supplement these acids. You'll find a number of companies make capsules that provide all the essential fatty acids you need each day. If you get one of these, you might not need to take a separate evening primrose capsule, because you'll already have a fair amount of GLA. But I like evening primrose oil for its effects on hair and skin, so I take one of those on top of a pill for the essential fatty acids.

· *Pycnogenol.* I almost didn't take this supplement since I don't think you should be swallowing something whose name you can't pronounce. Once I learned that it is "PICK-nog-e-nol," I felt a little better (and after I had been using it for several months, it did allow me to win a Scrabble game). Another strong antioxidant, pycnogenol helps stabilize collagen and maintain elastin—two critical proteins in skin, blood vessels, and muscle. It comes from plants, most notably pine bark and grape seeds. You can get some of the same effects if you eat buckets of cranberries or black currants, or drink gallons of green or black tea. Short of that, the only way to get this benefit is to take a daily supplement. You won't find it in any multivitamin, so a separate pill is the only choice here. The most highly touted in studies is that made from the French maritime pine bark (don't ask me why), so most health food stores stock that type. Nutritionists recommend between 25 and 100 milligrams a day. Not only is pycnogenol side effect free (according to the literature) but it is also water-soluble, so that any excess just gets passed through the body. However, being cautious as I am, I take the minimum amount, 25 milligrams, figuring it is better to get some of the protection without upping the dosage too high.

· *Garlic.* One of my favorite new supplements, garlic may seem simple enough to get in your diet, but not if you intend to have a lot of relationships up close and personal. Garlic breath is not a bother to most Europeans; I used to blissfully eat cloves cut into dishes and then wonder why most Americans grimaced or backed away from me, sometimes offering breath mints on the way out the door. So although I still eat garlic in my favorite foods, I also take a daily supplement of the odorless variety. In an impressive number of studies, garlic has shown benefits for the heart and nerves, enhancing the immune system, preventing and treating infection, and possibly lowering the risk of cancer. In one study the daily equivalent of one clove of garlic lowered cholesterol about nine points, enough to make a 20 percent difference in the long-term heart attack rate. It also helps reduce blood pressure and the likelihood of blood clots. Garlic is side effect free, and between 200 and 300 milligrams is the recommended dose.

· *Coenzyme Q$_{10}$* (fortunately, abbreviated by almost everyone as CQ$_{10}$). A vitaminlike substance related to vitamin E, CQ$_{10}$ is a powerful antioxidant that is found in all our organs and skin, but it diminishes with age. During menopause our stores get really depleted and can lead to a deficiency that results in greatly reduced energy and a slowing of the body's ability to rejuvenate and heal itself. Many athletes use CQ$_{10}$ to enhance performance. It is also used as an immune booster for treating heart disease in Japan, for helping the brain function properly, and for fighting premature aging; some people even recommend it for preventing cancer. You might get enough CQ$_{10}$ if you eat mackerel, sardines, and salmon. But if you have a more typical diet, you'll almost certainly benefit from a daily supplement. Although it is recommended in doses up to 100 milligrams, I take a conservative 30 milligrams a day. Again, you won't find this in your multivitamins. And girls, if you aren't persuaded by the possible health benefits of this wonderful supplement, you might be interested to learn that a recent study showed that people on a low-fat diet doubled their weight loss when they took CQ_{10}, compared with those in the study who did not take it.

· *Goldenseal.* This herb used to be one of the favorite cure-alls of the Cherokee Indians. It has won praise from medical researchers for helping the body bolster its immune system. I especially liked studies that showed it helps calm the digestive system, assists in good skin, and is a potent nerve tonic. Goldenseal allows the body to work at an internally slower pace than the treadmill speed with which we push ourselves in modern society. I take 100 milligrams daily of the extract and sometimes buy it bundled with another herb, echinacea, which has shown promise in warding off colds and the flu. I don't want to jinx myself, but since entering menopause and starting on my enhanced nutritional program, I haven't had a sick day, much less a cold. You should note, however, that if you suffer from low blood sugar, goldenseal lowers the blood sugar even more, so add it to your regimen only after asking your doctor.

That's the sum of my power boosters. Now to the more interesting and, for me, harder to decide upon list of supplements required specifically for dealing with the symptoms of menopause.

· *Calcium.* First and foremost, as I mentioned when discussing bone strength, is extra calcium. I take two pills a day. Sometimes if I am on the run, either traveling or doing errands all day around the city, I don't get a chance to take the second pill. Since I consider extra calcium a necessity, I usually carry a few of the new chocolate-flavored squares that contain 500 milligrams of calcium. There are several brands, sold in almost every general drugstore in the vitamin section; they're not only a clever way to get some calcium but a great mid-afternoon sweet for a guiltless and delicious 20 calories.

Each of my regular 600-milligram calcium softgels has 200 IU of vitamin D bundled in, which is important for the calcium's absorption. Another good trick to ensure that the calcium gets into your bones and isn't just passed through your body is to take some extra magnesium. It has a lot of benefits, but I like magnesium not only for its ability to speed calcium absorption but also for its role in mineralizing bones. Sugar and alcohol rob the body of magnesium, and if you don't have enough of this little wonder supplement, not only will your body lose calcium and potassium, but you can get other annoying problems, such as epileptic seizures, arteriosclerosis, impaired metabolism, mental confusion, depression, muscle cramps, and premature aging of the skin. If you eat a lot of alfalfa, kale, seaweed, whole grains, sunflower seeds, and unsulfured black molasses, you're probably getting enough magnesium from your diet. If you're like me and don't count those as regular items on your daily menu, you're best taking at least 250 milligrams—my dose—of magnesium daily, although some nutritionists suggest up to 750 milligrams.

· *Royal jelly.* No, I don't just like the "royal" moniker because I'm British, but you have to admit that a supplement with such an imperial-sounding name seems promising right off the bat. The jelly comes from worker bees, who feed it to the queen, hence its name. Actually, I use royal jelly primarily because of the studies that show it lowers cholesterol levels and fights arteriosclerosis; other evidence suggests it may have moderate antitumor properties. That covers some of the same ground as estrogen replacement. Although I didn't choose it because of its ability to fight hot flashes, some women swear that royal jelly has helped them beat those as well. Because there is a limited supply of natural royal jelly, it tends to be expensive. Try to find 500-milligram pills and take one daily.

· *Ginkgo biloba.* You've probably heard of this natural herb, which is harvested from the leaves of trees that grow primarily in China and parts of the United States, for its promise in aiding Alzheimer's patients. More than three hundred scientific studies have cited it as one of the most promising brain foods in decades, with patients usually showing cognitive improvements from a couple of weeks to three months after they start taking it. That's one of the chief reasons I added ginkgo to my nutritional regimen, especially because menopause tends to cause some women to experience cloudiness or confusion. This can be just a passing phase of extra-forgetfulness. I figured ginkgo would help. It works by enhancing energy production in the brain, and by increasing the glucose absorbed by brain cells, it actually improves the transmission of nerve signals. The faster those signals are transferred, the better your memory. And when I began doing a little research, I found studies that also showed ginkgo to promise help for other symptoms of menopause—including depression and migraines—as well as one of the longer-term possible effects of reduced estrogen, arteriosclerosis.

The use of ginkgo has been traced back almost five thousand years to Chinese herbal medicine. Since ginkgo makes circulation more efficient, you might not want to use it if you are planning surgery, as it could increase your bleeding. Cut it out for a week or so beforehand, just as you would vitamin E. Also, this is one supplement best not taken with your coffee. Ginkgo expands the blood vessels, whereas caffeine shrinks them, so the two work against each other and could give you a headache. Nutritionists recommend between 120 and 320 milligrams a day of the extract. Being my cautious self, I take 120 milligrams, broken into two 60-milligram doses, one in the morning and one in the evening. There are very few reported side effects; a small number of people get either headaches or a mildly upset stomach when first trying ginkgo. I did not experience any problems.

· *Soy isoflavones.* You know that I added tofu to some of my salads, so you might be wondering why I am also taking a soy supplement. It's because you would have to eat a *lot* of tofu to get all the soy you need, and after a while, no matter how clever a cook you are, you run out of ways to make tofu tasty. There are some nights you just can't stomach it anymore, and if you're traveling you might not come across a restaurant with tofu anywhere between Salt Lake City and Detroit. In these cases, and on days when you don't want to look at any more tofu or eat another GeniSoy bar, soy isoflavones are the perfect remedy.

Why is soy so important? Its isoflavones enhance your immune system while lowering cholesterol levels. By helping to regulate the hormones we still produce, isoflavones may also reduce the risk of hormone-dependent cancers, such as breast and prostate cancer.

And of course, I was attracted to soy because stomach acids convert the isoflavones into compounds that have mild estrogen effects, easing menopausal symptoms for many women without the baggage of estrogen. Although isoflavones have an estrogenlike effect, they are not hormones. One of the studies that helped convince me was of fifty-eight menopausal women who experienced an average of fourteen hot flashes per week. They supplemented their diets with either wheat flour or soy flour every day for three months, and the soy-flour group reduced their hot flashes by over 40 percent.

So unless you are eating a lot of soy in foods like tofu, tempeh, soy milk, miso, or soy sauce, you'd better get soy in a good supplement. The interesting thing about soy is that if you don't consume any, and don't supplement your diet with it, you won't be deficient in it. It's not like one of the body's required vitamins or minerals. But if you don't consume soy or take a supplement, you won't get any of the benefits either.

As for the right dosage, no one knows the ideal intake. Asian women, who experience far fewer menopausal side effects than those of us in the West, eat a lot of soy. I take 50 milligrams of the soy extract, which approximates what the average Asian woman consumes daily. The only caveat (beyond possible allergy to soy products, which should make you avoid all of this) is that soy contains a compound that can interfere with mineral absorption. So if you want to be especially careful, you might take your soy supplement separate from your mineral-containing multivitamin.

· *Ginseng.* Another of my new supplements, ginseng has been touted by nutritionists as an aid for everything from Alzheimer's disease to chronic fatigue syndrome. Dating back some two thousand years in Chinese medicine, ginseng was used to battle infections as well as colds and flu. It was also believed to provide energy and vitality. In modern times ginseng's ability to increase stamina and endurance led Soviet Olympic athletes to use it as a training enhancer. After the Chernobyl nuclear accident, many Russians were given ginseng as part of the program to counteract the effects of radiation fallout.

I wasn't planning to enter the Olympics or get exposed to a toxic dose of radiation, so my attraction to ginseng was different. Ginseng seemed to me a good addition since it not only combats harmful toxins in the body but also enhances the work done by the adrenal glands, even when we are under great stress. Since the adrenals take over hormone production after our ovaries shut down in menopause, it's wise to give them as much nutritional support as possible. Another attraction of ginseng is its ability to improve the flow of oxygen to muscles, letting exercisers work out longer and recover quicker from those workouts. Known to nutritionists as an adaptogen, ginseng is an all-around rejuvenator, helping your body adapt to the sometimes stressful changes brought on by menopause.

How much should you use? Nutritionists recommend between 1000 and 2000 milligrams a day of the dry powdered root, in a capsule. I take 1000 milligrams. As for side effects, they are very mild, with a few people reporting diarrhea when first adding ginseng to their daily regimen, and others having trouble sleeping if they take it too close to bedtime. Also, there are different types of ginseng, and users who get far more involved in the details than I do will debate for hours the relative merits and disadvantages of each—Korean, Chinese, American, or Siberian. I settled the debate for myself in the most Solomonic manner I could find: One company, Herbal World, makes 1000-milligram capsules that have equal amounts of each of the four types of ginseng and, as a bonus, includes 200 milligrams of pure royal jelly. Thus, this product offers the added benefit of combining several pills into one easy-to-remember capsule.

The final supplement I take is one of my favorites, in part because it combines into a single capsule seven herbs. Called Change-O-Life by Nature's Way, it provides equal doses, in a 440-milligram capsule, of black cohosh root, sarsaparilla root, licorice root, blessed thistle herb, squaw vine herb, and false unicorn root. It also has some Siberian ginseng. Black cohosh, one of the most popular menopausal herbs in Europe, helps maintain hormonal balance on lower estrogen levels, reduces hot flashes, helps with bone density loss, and lessens water retention. Sarsaparilla root—long used as a flavoring agent in root beer—has a very mild progesteronelike effect but without the side effects. It boosts energy and helps the skin stay elastic and vibrant. Licorice has an estrogenic effect without producing any estrogen, so it helps with many menopausal symptoms, such as hot flashes (but beware if you have high blood pressure—licorice can elevate it). Blessed thistle helps with bone density and calms the digestive system. Squaw vine is a uterine and ovarian tonic, relieving bouts of cramping or bloating. False unicorn root also has an estrogenic effect and helps maintain a balance of the hormones your body still produces.

Just because these are herbs doesn't mean they aren't powerful. Since some of them have estrogenic effects, and although the level of estrogen is very low—about 1 percent as strong as regular estrogen—I don't want to take them in megadoses but prefer the small doses of each in this single pill. These herbs are often known as balancers since they have the ability not only to raise low estrogen levels but also to lower high levels. And they seem to work better, according to some of the literature, if they are digested together. Sure, you could buy all six in separate pills, but that seems to me to be a lot of extra work. Pamper yourself, and get the single capsule that knocks off all six at once. Your body will thank you.

. . .

Finally, if you know something about herbs and nutritional supplements, you might wonder why I left out certain ones that are often recommended for women in menopause. For instance, among herbs often touted are vitex (chaste tree), yarrow, dandelion, motherwort, and dong quai. Also, among vitamins, some women swear by linseed oil for their skin. Other women who have family histories of breast cancer add gamma oryzanol, a component of rice bran oil, to their diets. Some swear it reduces menopausal symptoms and even lowers cholesterol, while not adversely affecting their hormone levels. I did try many of these substances, for at least six weeks at a time, and noticed no difference whether they were in or out of my routine. So instead of just adding a supplement to my daily intake because some book recommended it, I have tried to winnow my list to the bare necessities. The herbs and vitamins that I did not use may be wonderful for someone else. I am convinced, after my research, that there is no single program that fits every woman. You need to experiment a little to discover which supplements work for you, and particularly how the group you are taking work synergistically on your body. We are all born with individual biological blueprints that determine not only our nutritional requirements but also how different nutrients and doses react in our bodies.

So much also depends on lifestyle. Maybe my regimen wouldn't work so well if I still smoked, or didn't exercise, or ate a lot of saturated fat. None of the elements of our lives—including nutritional supplements—can be considered in a vacuum. So if you find that dong quai alleviates your hot flashes, great. Just because it didn't work for me doesn't mean it won't for you. Taken in moderation, these herbs and supplements will not harm you. And if you discover the right combination to alleviate your symptoms, they will definitely change your life for the better.

THIRTEEN

Sex Once More

ONE of the aspects of my relationship with Gerald that was particularly healthy was our sex life. We had been together for sixteen years before I was diagnosed as menopausal. During those years, our sex life thrived, in part because we imposed no routine or set schedule, just let it remain spontaneous. Sure, there were periods, as in any marriage, when we weren't as active because some book deadline loomed and neither of us could get much energy or enthusiasm for anything at night but crashing out. But there would be other times when we would behave like newlyweds and wonder what spell had settled over us. We were similar; despite having become the best of friends and spending most days together, we had never lost our physical attraction to each other.

That is precisely why it was so unusual when for about six months sex became the farthest thing from my mind. I just had no desire. It wasn't anything to do with Gerald; it was my own problem, but I didn't feel really compelled to fix it because the whole idea of sex simply didn't interest me. Gerald and I have always been very affectionate with each other, and I enjoyed cuddling and hugging in bed as much as ever, but it never got beyond that. I blamed my initial blasé attitude on deadlines and stress, but eventually it was pretty clear to both of us that something unusual was going on. Gerald was amazingly patient during all of this, although I think he might have been quite frustrated at times. But the saving grace for our relationship was that he never took my lack of interest personally. When he found out it was a result of menopause, he only hoped that this would be the symptom that I would most rapidly and effectively treat with my new regimen. At one point he gave me an article that talked about how good sex is for all of us, how it stimulates a woman's hormones, releases tension, calms us, boosts the immune system, and relieves headaches and maybe even arthritis. I remember laughing loudly as I read it.

"What's so funny?" Gerald asked.

"You don't have to convince me that sex is good for me." I smiled and shook my head. "I'm sure this is all true. But I'd like to feel I could get back in the groove for a simpler reason—that it just feels great."

"I guess I might have been overselling it," he admitted.

After a little research, I learned that a loss of libido is not unusual for menopausal women. Doctors blame one of our declining hormones, testosterone. But I did not subscribe to the belief of some physicians that loss of desire is a natural development as we age. Since I had already considered and rejected testosterone replacement, I had to look for natural alternatives. One nutritionist recommended extra supplements of magnesium, zinc, and vitamin B_6. But since I already took those as part of my general nutritional program, and I didn't seem to be jumping on my husband at every other opportunity, I figured something else might be required. I did up my B_6 from 50 milligrams to 100, since it is essential for the conversion of serotonin, which is a prerequisite for a healthy libido. I was pleased to discover quite late in my research that sarsaparilla, which was already in my "change of life" supplement, stimulates the little production of testosterone we have during menopause, thereby helping to boost a flagging libido.

I do not believe that any herbs are natural aphrodisiacs, although some less than reputable nutritionists would disagree. And I did not suddenly start eating oysters and other foods that some people claim put them in the mood. A girlfriend told me that aromatherapy—the use of scented essential oils—worked for her, especially lavender and pumpkin pie. I tried it, but all that happened was I got hungry. Not quite what I was looking for.

Although I thought it was a myth that once a woman hits menopause sex is over, I must say I was a little worried. And I had none of the obvious reasons for my lack of desire, such as reduced self-esteem or a negative body image. If anything, both had improved with my more rigorous exercise and diet. I began to wonder if anything was wrong with me, since I didn't feel the way I should.

It took me considerable time to stop fretting over it.

Since Gerald wasn't pushing me, I realized I could relax about the situation. It was a very strange development, but once I stopped worrying about why I wasn't interested in sex, my desire slowly started returning. It was almost the same as one of those nights when you can't fall asleep so instead you look at the bedside clock every half hour and fret about how tired you'll be the following morning; all that worry about how little sleep you are getting is guaranteed to keep you awake. I think the constant fretting about my lack of sex drive, and my sometimes forced attempts to "get in the mood," actually further diminished my interest.

Beyond the psychological change of just letting go, I was also half a year into my supplement, exercise, and food program when I noticed that I was starting to feel more like my old self. I think it is also likely that my new regimen helped balance my system and stabilize my hormone production, even testosterone at reduced levels. But I really can't pick one thing that made a difference. All I know with any certainty is that one night, after getting home from a dinner party at which I'd had a glass of wine or two (but certainly wasn't tipsy), I looked at Gerald and strongly felt the urge that had been missing. That night was a turning point, putting us back on track. But for the very same reason that I couldn't explain to you, much less to myself, why my interest had suddenly waned, I also couldn't tell you why it happened to return that night.

I was fortunate not to have the vaginal dryness that afflicts many women in menopause. While it is easily treatable with over-the-counter topical creams, vaginal dryness probably contributes more than any other symptom to the stereotype of the postmenopausal woman as "drying up." On this count, I may have benefited from my increased soy intake, extra vitamin E, and daily doses of black cohosh, beta-carotene, evening primrose oil, and essential fatty acids. Many nutritionists recommend these supplements for women suffering from this symptom, and some state unequivocally that they boost the sex hormone production of the adrenal glands.

Now, girls, don't get me wrong—I haven't become a nymphomaniac by any stretch of the imagination. But I am back to enjoying an active sex life with my dear husband, and that feels right for us. I think part of getting over my lackluster libido was also adjusting, physically and psychologically, to this midlife passage. Once I began feeling that I had taken back control of what was happening to my body, I started to feel better about sex as well. In the end, my brain was the most important sex organ, because it ultimately controlled the way I viewed sex and my desire to have it.

I'm not sure what would have happened if my husband had harangued me during those months, but I am pretty sure it would have worsened my worry about my lack of desire and might well have postponed any return to normalcy. I think what you need to remember is that if you pass through menopause and suddenly lose the desire for sex, it's really OK. It is just one of those things that might happen. You and your mate need to communicate and be patient with each other. It also helps if you receive some encouragement that this is not your fault but rather just a phase. With this approach, I think you will be pleasantly surprised that some real ardor can again be yours.

FOURTEEN

Beating the Blues

DIDN'T know how lucky I had been to never have really experienced blue days, serious anxiety, or mild depression before I entered menopause. The more I spoke to women my age, the more I realized that this general malaise, which can settle over a day with no rhyme or reason, is much more common than I ever imagined. A few years back, for instance, when I was still suffering migraine headaches, I had been put on a new prescription. Sometimes, when girlfriends said that they also suffered from severe headaches, I'd mention my medication, which was helping me. Most of them recognized the new pill, which had been widely discussed in the press. "Oh, no," I'd invariably be told, "I can't use that, since I'm on antidepressants."

Once my general practitioner commented on how "up" I always seemed. When I assured him that I did have my off days, he shook his head. "Trisha, people confide in me as a doctor. They often talk about very personal things. You'd be shocked how many people suffer from real depression. You're one of the most up people I know. I'm sure your down days are better than most people's good days."

My blue days may have been mild compared with those of some people, and they were admittedly infrequent, but since I was so unaccustomed to feeling down, they were for me memorable and upsetting. On those days when I felt out of sorts, I had little enthusiasm for doing much and felt as though I were on an emotional roller coaster. At other times, I would just be irritable. I'd warn Gerald that for some reason I was feeling blue and if I snapped at him it was nothing that he had said or done. Once I forewarned him, he would tread very carefully with me that day, and such communication almost always helped us avoid a misunderstanding about my behavior. That kind of openness with your mate is critical. It felt better, somehow, telling Gerald that I was out of sorts. I wasn't embarrassed by it, since it was something over which I initially had no control. But letting him in on my state of mind made me feel I wasn't alone.

My research pointed out that hormonal changes don't actually induce the blues. But they do change the body's natural balance, so something that might not ordinarily bother us at all can become quite upsetting. Also, there are some typical culprits for adding to this malaise, such as alcohol and cigarettes—both depressants. I'm a nonsmoker who has a glass of white wine several times a week, so I figured that wasn't my problem. Nutritional deficiencies—especially vitamins B_{12} and C, folic acid, and niacin—can lead to depression, but I doubted that I was short of any of these. The more reasonable explanation seemed to be that some women just find mood swings common as hormones drastically change.

Finally, from my own experience, I am fairly positive that the blues that come with menopause result more from the changes our bodies are undergoing than from any measurement of how we feel about ourselves and life in general. While our emotional state will obviously affect the degree to which we are bothered by hormone shifts, there is a physical element to this passage that cannot be waved away with platitudes and positive thinking. On days when I felt down, I would make a list of all I had to be happy about— I've got a great life, and I don't take it for granted but am very thankful for it. But that wouldn't lift me. That's what made the feeling so unusual. It was almost as though my spirit had a mind of its own and on some days it just decided to be blue. This was, at least for me, a very troubling sensation. It almost made me feel a stranger in my own skin.

St. John's wort, an herb that is wildly popular in Europe and becoming more widespread in the United States, helps treat symptoms of anxiety and depression. While some prescription mood elevators have a long list of side effects, St. John's wort has virtually none. But I didn't want to adopt an herb that was targeted just to this symptom, because it was not a constant problem. Using a steady herb supplement to treat a symptom that was infrequently present seemed to me a bit of overkill. Initially, I put St. John's wort on my maybe list, something to return to if I did not see improvement.

But I never got a chance to try St. John's wort. That's because once I had spent a few months with my battery of nutritional supplements, my healthier diet, and my more vigorous exercise routine, I noticed that my blue days seemed fewer and farther between. Before starting my new program, I went through months when I would have at least one down day a week. During the first three months of my program, when I kept a loose sort of daily diary marking the physical and mental changes I noticed, I listed a dozen days when I felt out of sorts and down in the dumps. In the next three months, that was down to two days. I wish I could pinpoint a single nutrient or food group that made the difference.

There are several possible explanations. Ginkgo biloba, which I was taking as a guardian against potential memory and concentration problems, is also cited in some studies as having mild antidepressant benefits. Ginseng, also part of my routine, is sometimes promoted as having a calming effect. In my multivitamin I was getting extra doses of B_5 and choline, which are precursors for brain chemicals that can cause depression if they are too low. Also, more vigorous exercise makes the brain release endorphins, the body's own pain-relieving and antidepressant agents. Exercise and acupuncture are known to stimulate endorphin production, and since I wasn't using acupuncture, I figured that only my new gym routine could be responsible for help on that front.

It could be that the ginkgo, ginseng, and exercise in combination helped to lift my mild case of the blues. But I also think that part of the solution was acknowledging the physical symptoms I had tried to deny. My hot flashes, irritability, headaches, and loss of libido took away some of my confidence. I can't prove it, but I have a sneaking suspicion that, given my preference for being in control, all the uncertainty surrounding my menopausal symptoms and what I would do about them helped put me into my occasional funk. Part of getting past it was achieving a positive new attitude about how I was progressing through menopause and where I wanted to be when I finished with it. With my own program, I had a sense of accomplishment and purpose. That helped me feel myself again.

I have no doubt that many women are bothered by more serious depression than my flirting with the blues, and if you are prone to depression even before menopause, the hormone changes could definitely worsen it for you. In that case, St. John's wort would be a good first remedy. If I had had to choose one supplement if my mood problem had persisted, it would have been that herb. Certainly, St. John's wort would come much earlier on my option list than Prozac or one of the more powerful prescription antidepressants.

Besides the blues, several other symptoms also pretty much disappeared after my new program had been in place for a couple of months. One thing I was glad to lose were my headaches. I have long been a headache sufferer, but they seemed to peak in intensity and frequency just before and at the beginning of menopause. I couldn't blame them all on everyday stress. But during the past year to eighteen months, while I still occasionally get a headache, they seem to have been much less frequent than in previous decades, and they go quicker if I take some aspirin or Tylenol. Black cohosh, one of my regular supplements, is used by some nutritionists to treat headaches that result from anxiety. It might have contributed to my relief, but I also think that my cleaner diet and better exercise helped. For those of you undergoing menopause and still fighting headaches, the other herbs that had been on my short list, but that I never experimented with once my headaches dissipated, included feverfew, which helps headaches that result from stress; valerian, for headaches from nervous tension; and Avena sativa if the headache might be from overwork or depression. Any of these added to your daily regimen might make your headaches just a bad memory.

Another menopause experience that disappeared was my heart palpitations. My heart would start racing, and while sometimes this would come just before a hot flash, often it was on its own. Then I read a little about heart palpitations and discovered that they result from out-of-balance hormones and are related to the same mechanisms that produce hot flashes. Smoking and heavy drinking can worsen this symptom, but those weren't my culprits. But once again, after staying on my new program for about two months, I noticed that I hadn't had a heart-racing attack. Much nutritional literature points out that extra doses of vitamin E, calcium, and magnesium are helpful for minimizing heart palpitations. These were all vitamins whose dosages I had sharply increased. Also, two of my other supplements, CQ_{10} and ginkgo biloba, help supply both energy to the heart cells and oxygen to the blood and heart, two features that should allow the heart to relax. Again, I'm not sure what the specific trick was, or if it was several things working synergistically, but I do know that I haven't had a bout of rapid heartbeats in the past two years.

I know this might sound strange, but I didn't immediately notice that some symptoms, like the rapid heartbeats and headaches, were gone. It was just that for some time I felt fine. Then one day Gerald commented that it seemed like a long time since I had suffered from a headache, and when we really thought about how long, it was clear that something good had happened to me. Of course, being superstitious, I was convinced that Gerald's mentioning of it would curse me with an instant headache, but one did not immediately appear. It was the same with the heart palpitations. And one day, when I went to chronicle what had happened to my hot flashes, I realized that this symptom had also gone. For me, that is part of the power of an all-natural approach to menopause. If you have a program that pampers the mind and body, you'll just find yourself feeling fine and not concentrating on each of the admittedly aggravating symptoms of menopause. Before you know it, you'll stop thinking about them because they'll no longer be there. Symptom-free menopause is indeed wonderful.

FIFTEEN

Testing for Success

THAT first year of full menopause passed remarkably quickly. Months had been consumed with reading everything I could find, and then the trial and error of introducing herbal remedies, trying vitamin and mineral supplements, changing my beauty regimen, adapting to my new way of eating, and getting used to my more rigorous exercise program. By that time I started to feel like myself again—in other words, feeling premenopausal, except for the fact that I no longer had a period. By the end of that first year, my occasional blue days were a thing of the past, my sex drive had slowly but steadily returned, and I felt stronger than I had in years. At least from the outside, my program had worked. I was in better shape than ever; at almost ten pounds less, I certainly felt good, and I also had greater endurance and strength. No longer was I winded when climbing a few flights of stairs or tired after walking half the day around Manhattan. My body tone—tighter muscles and no sagging skin—was better than when I started. The best test, standing undressed in front of a mirror with an overhead fluorescent light—you know, girls, the type of dressing room in which department stores make you try on swimsuits—was still not something I relished, but it was no longer cause for an anxiety attack.

I knew the true measure of my success was not just how I felt and looked, although the two go hand in hand since our self-esteem and happiness are partially dependent on how satisfied we are with how we age. The real test was now due—my full annual physical exam by my general practitioner, followed by another bone density test to see how my bones had fared a year after my body had virtually stopped producing estrogen. Comparing the results with those of the prior year would tell me whether my program was helping my heart and bones.

When I arrived at my regular doctor's office, he commented on the way I looked. "You don't look like menopause," he said, smiling, as we began the exam. It reminded me of the question I had posed to Gerald nearly a year ago: "Does this look like menopause?"

The test results that came in that day and the following week gave me great satisfaction. My sitting pulse rate had dropped from 92 to 57 a minute. My cholesterol was down from 197 to 167, and my ratio of good to bad cholesterol had actually improved, now a very low 2:1. On the stress test conducted on a treadmill, I went faster and farther without getting my heart rate anywhere near the level it was the year before.

"Trisha, you are in excellent shape for someone in her thirties, much less someone approaching fifty," my doctor told me as he reviewed the paperwork. I left his office that day on cloud nine, feeling as though I had just gotten the medical stamp of approval on my natural menopausal program. Only my bone density test was still to come.

While in San Francisco for a few weeks visiting my mother-in-law, I again went through the nearly thirty-minute DEXA procedure, a low-level X-ray exam that precisely measures bone density. It took nearly a week to discover that those results were even better than my baseline, which my gynecologist had deemed "superb."

I knew how good the results were when my gynecologist, who had counseled me strongly that I was in trouble if I did not adopt hormone replacement therapy, at first thought he had the wrong test results on my summary sheet. He had expected to see a decline, and the improvement really surprised him. It was the first meeting we had had in quite a while in which he did not suggest that I move on to hormones.

He studied the reports from my regular doctor carefully, then looked up at me. "Trisha, whatever you are doing . . ."

I was prepared to hear some warning.

". . . just keep doing it. It's working, and you're doing fine."

It was the final professional pat on the back I wanted. And it pleased me because, despite our disagreement over whether I should take hormones, I otherwise adore my gynecologist, and I trust him implicitly on many questions regarding my health. Now it felt as though we could get on with our doctor-patient relationship. That was comforting.

It's hard to explain how uplifting those test results were. I had been eager to discover what my homegrown program was doing for my heart and bones. Now I had the answer: They had gotten better with the rest of me. Any woman on hormone replacement therapy must be equally pleased when she feels like herself again and gets good news on her health. But for me there was the additional benefit that I had accomplished this not only on my own but also without anything that added to my fear of breast cancer. It was liberating to get good medical news without any looming worry.

When I got home I announced my gynecologist's endorsement to Gerald.

"I expected no less," he said, crossing the room to a large closet.

"Oh, you probably had your doubts that this would work so well," I said to him. "Admit it."

"Nope. I had faith," he insisted. Inside the closet, he reached under a group of sweaters and pulled out something that he had apparently hidden away. With a flourish he swung around and unfurled a white T-shirt. Emblazoned across the front was a caricature of St. George slaying the dragon. Under the drawing, in Gothic script, it read, TRISHA: MENOPAUSE SLAYER.

"You earned it," Gerald said.

I must say I agreed.

SIXTEEN

Freedom and Power

AS a society, Americans are obsessed with youth. So instead of approaching menopause as an opportunity for change and growth, we are conditioned to view it as the end of our reproductive ability and hence our sexual attractiveness. Instead of a new start, it is pigeonholed as the end of a vibrant phase of life. Even the word *menopause,* derived from Greek words that mean "monthly" and "cause to cease," is filled with the connotation that this is an end, not a beginning.

But I firmly believe that menopause holds much more promise than that, and is a time of transition that offers each of us a chance to reevaluate our relationships, what we are doing with our lives, and how we are taking care of our physical and emotional health. It gives us a chance at rebirth. The same way that puberty presented us with tremendous change and immense possibilities as we entered young adulthood, menopause promises that we are wise enough to enjoy our most satisfying years in this last long stretch of our lives. Menopause is certainly not a time to be feared, as many medical practitioners cast it. And all of us as women should refuse to be worn down by society's devaluation of us once we pass menopause.

Although menopause seems foreboding to most women in the United States, there are many cultures where it is welcomed. Postmenopausal Indian women can enter Hindu temples and participate in rituals. Thai women mark the occasion with a celebration and gain new respect for having attained a status of experience and wisdom. In central Asia women welcome menopause as a movement into the most enlightened part of their lives. Women in those cultures where menopause is viewed positively often report far fewer symptoms than do those of us in the West. That leaves me with little doubt that, while menopause is undeniably a biological event, social and cultural factors are very important in affecting the way we react to this change.

I know that the symptoms that usually accompany menopause can be quite troubling, but my experience also shows that those symptoms are not an inevitable part of this change, and that a holistic approach—natural medications and supplements combined with an active, healthy, and balanced lifestyle—offers a safe alternative to the traditional medical approach of hormone replacement therapy.

Postmenopausal zest is a phrase coined by the anthropologist Margaret Mead, who discovered a renewed productivity and love of life in her fifties. Hindus call it *dharma,* establishing a personal connection with the divine. Some scientists contend that once menstruation ends a woman's testosterone-to-estrogen ratio rises, enhancing vitality and confidence. Whatever one calls it or however one explains it, I know the phenomenon is real.

Some women in menopause might say, "I don't feel like my old self." That's often interpreted to mean something is wrong. But that feeling of change should be embraced. The menopausal woman is unlikely to feel like her old self, because she isn't. She is a new woman. It's not called the change of life for nothing.

I now realize that when I was told I was in menopause I went through not only some denial but also some fear that my best years were over, that I was entering a difficult period when my body and mind might start to betray me. And the more I read and spoke with other women, the more I found that these are remarkably common feelings. Yet I believe that how you confront these fears and doubts has much to do with how you will pass through menopause. Instead of allowing them to cripple me, or to hold me back, I tackled this experience as a new challenge, one that I was determined to master. It was great to have the support of Gerald, but in the end it had to be my passage. Girls, as much love and support as you have, there is something solitary about this change, and there will be times when you just need to sit by yourself and work through whatever happens to be bothering you.

For those of you who do opt for estrogen replacement—and I know many women who do and are quite pleased—I think that is great. But don't just take the prescription because your gynecologist has written one. Do a little research and really think about whether it is right for you. Be an informed consumer. You all know a girlfriend who has spent more time looking for a new hairdresser than deciding whether to start hormone replacement therapy. Just apply the same zeal and control that you do in so many other aspects of your life.

And most important, remember there are choices out there beyond what our doctors might tell us. Traditional medicine is remarkably narrow in its focus, and menopause is a time when we need not only to treat the physical but also to nurture the spiritual and emotional.

My passage through menopause has filled me with a sense of empowerment and independence. It served as a gateway to a time of physical, spiritual, and emotional growth that I never expected. It also meant freedom: no more menstrual cramps, or PMS, or monthly bouts with swollen and tender breasts, and no more birth control. I felt invigorated. I had taken control by ensuring that I entered this new phase of my life in great condition and on my own terms.

Although blood tests for FSH and estrogen levels are pretty good indicators of whether you are in menopause, most doctors don't confirm it until you have passed a full year since your last period. For a couple of months before I hit that milestone, I thought it would be only right to mark that anniversary with something that I would remember. As good fortune would have it, we visited Paris that week, having just finished a trip to see my mother in London. We were only in the City of Lights for a few days, but I set aside the morning of my official marker of menopause. I left with Gerald on the métro for the Left Bank. He had to visit a friend who was leaving the city that day, and I planned to meet him in a couple of hours for lunch. It is unusual for us to do almost anything separately, but this seemed right on my own.

My destination was the Sacré-Coeur, a fabulous Roman- and Byzantine-style basilica that sits atop a hill with an imposing view of neighboring Montmartre and all of Paris. My choice was unusual since I am Jewish and thus obviously not prone to think of Catholic churches as sites for special days. But this journey carried extra meaning. When I was a child, my aunt and uncle used to take me for holidays to Paris. My uncle, an amateur but earnest painter, found the artists' quarter of Montmartre one of his favorite stops. As a remarkably shy child (those who know me now find it nearly impossible to imagine I was once a retiring wallflower), I used to cringe at the gauntlet of local artists who would incessantly ask to draw my picture. Montmartre for me was not a charming and beguiling backwater district but rather the most nerve-racking part of my visit.

Now I would revisit that site of such childhood trepidation as a woman who had passed into a final and very different phase of life. And Sacré-Coeur was important for a different reason. I knew that two wealthy Parisians had built it at the turn of the century to commemorate France's victory in two wars against Germany. I liked the fact that it was dedicated to perseverance and victory, which I had experienced in my battle with menopause and my doctor's advice about hormones. My uncle, although he had little time for churches, loved that one of his favorite artists, Maurice Utrillo, never tired of drawing and painting there. As a child, I had once visited this place, and I remembered trying unsuccessfully to climb the hundreds of stone steps that curve up at dizzying angles inside the bell tower, promising spectacular vistas from narrow walkways that adorn the outside of the church. Now I was determined to make that climb and see the panorama that had escaped me as a youngster.

Montmartre had definitely changed in the more than thirty years since I had last seen it. Although it retained its physical charms—its small-village atmosphere and narrow cobbled streets—it seemed that most of the artists and writers had long since left. As I strolled through the old square, Place du Tertre, the quick-portrait artists who lay in wait for the mobs of eager tourists that ascend the hill daily again bombarded me. This time I merely shook my head no and smiled. I wasn't sure whether the place had really changed—it seemed smaller, tackier, and not in the least intimidating—or whether the changes had been in me. I thought back to the little girl who used to be so nervous on these same streets. That girl who had no confidence was now the woman who was marking a whole new phase of her life. It felt comforting, and I gathered a certain strength as I continued walking up the hill, my pace quickening and my senses heightened.

If Montmartre had seemed somehow less than I remembered, Sacré-Coeur did not disappoint; it was still imposing and architecturally impressive. I went to the tiny side entrance and bought a ticket that both allowed me into the eerie underground crypts and gave me permission to climb the tower staircase.

I was early, one of the first people inside the basilica when it opened. I walked quickly through the vaulted crypts, the sound of my heels echoing off the stone walls. Then I arrived at the beginning of the staircase. I had remembered it as tiny, and this was one instance in which my memory had not failed me. Sacré-Coeur's stone stairs are narrow and wind at sharp curves inside a dimly lit tower. Every thirty steps or so, a slit cut into the stone wall lets some sunlight in. Then, occasionally, the staircase opens out onto part of the exterior of the grand church, and after you walk across some ridiculously narrow gangway, you continue your climb inside another tower.

I effortlessly tackled that first long flight of stairs. I was back to conquer what had beaten me as a child, and I seemed to have more strength and energy with each step. I was commemorating my anniversary with my own little endurance test. I could hear my quickened breath, and feel my heart pounding faster. There was a slight ache in my legs, but I didn't slow down. That ache, the perspiration, the labored breathing, they were the signs of vitality that I wanted to embrace.

When I had arrived that morning, thick clouds were moving into Paris. Rain had been forecast by midday. But the storm came earlier than expected. When I walked out of the first tower, I was standing along a narrow parapet that faced back to Montmartre. The sky had turned a menacing gray, as if early night had suddenly fallen. Large stone gargoyles projected out near my feet. And as I surveyed the beauty of the city, there was a torrential downpour, the type of cloudburst that soaks everything before leaving only some quick puddles as evidence of its fleeting but powerful appearance. When the first drops hit me, I did not run inside, as would have been my normal reaction. Instead, I stayed outside, the rain pelting all around, completely drenching me. As a child I had loved the rain and, to my mother's consternation, would get sopping wet before heading home and dripping all over her white carpeting. "You're a strange child," she'd admonish me as she vigorously towel-dried me. It didn't seem strange to me. I just liked the rain.

And on that day, perched over the gargoyles that mythically protect Sacré-Coeur, I again reveled in the rain. I stretched out my arms and turned up my face to embrace it. In part I was embracing myself, the new child that I had found, this one discovered in the most unlikely of places during the past year, menopause. The little girl who had so timidly walked the narrow streets below seemed a very distant memory. The rain that pelted my face and matted my hair and soaked my clothes was a force of nature, no less mysterious or wonderful to me than what I had discovered nature had built into my own body. Menopause. It had been a surprisingly wonderful journey.

N OW, ladies, you probably can tell by this point
that I'm someone who not only likes to be in control of the events in her life but also likes to make decisions
with lots of information under her belt. The program I developed through trial and error for my own menopause has
obviously worked very well for me, but I'm not a doctor, so
don't try something unless you talk first to a physician,
preferably one who is up-to-date on natural alternatives to
traditional medical choices. I don't know if my regimen
will work for other women, but I would be quite pleased if
many women just picked up a little help from it—maybe a
supplement that will lessen hot flashes, or some tricks to
strengthen bones, or a renewed desire to exercise and re-
claim a figure thought to have been lost forever. If that happens, then this book was a worthwhile endeavor.

I think those of you in menopause will understand, and

those approaching will soon know, that while the physical symptoms are the ones usually spoken about, the overall changes coupled with society's view of menopause can also shake our self-confidence and affect our emotional balance. At least for me, and I'm sure for many other women who like to think we control the direction of our lives, making one's own decisions about how to cope with menopause is a start toward getting in the right frame of mind for entering this next phase of life.

Let's bring menopause out of the closet. Let's not put future generations of women in the position I found myself, unable to get most acquaintances to even acknowledge that they'd been through it. There should be no shame associated with menopause. I'm proud of it. It has given me an edge that I only wish I could bottle and provide to other women.

We're all going to share this passage at some point. So approach it positively and make it work for you. Hopefully, one day American women will be honored at menopause by a culture that acknowledges we have paid our dues and have the wisdom of experience to make some of our most important contributions to family and society. And if you do it right for only one person, do it for yourself. Empower yourself through change.

BOOKS

Brody, Jane. *Jane Brody's Nutrition Book.* New York: W. W. Norton, 1981.

Brown, Ellen, and Lynn Walker. *Menopause and Estrogen: Natural Alternatives to Hormone Replacement Therapy.* Berkeley, CA: Frog, 1996.

Cabot, Sandra. *Smart Medicine for Menopause: Hormone Replacement Therapy and Its Natural Alternatives.* Garden City Park, NY: Avery Publishing, 1995.

Crawford, Amanda McQuade. *The Herbal Menopause Book: Herbs, Nutrition, and Other Natural Therapies.* Freedom, CA: Crossing Press, 1996.

Dean, Carolyn. *Menopause Naturally: A Wide Range of Natural Therapies to Help Women Through This Challenging Passage.* New Canaan, CT: Keats Publishing, 1995.

Glenville, Marilyn. *Natural Choices for Menopause.* New York: St. Martin's Press, 1997.

Goldstein, Steven R., and Laurie Ashner. *The Estrogen Alternative: What Every Woman Needs to Know About Hormone Replacement Therapy and SERMS, the New Estrogen Substitutes.* New York: G. P. Putnam's Sons, 1998.

Griffith, H. Winter. *Complete Guide to Vitamins, Minerals, and Supplements.* Tucson, AZ: Fisher Books, 1988.

Ito, Dee. *Without Estrogen: Natural Remedies for Menopause and Beyond.* New York: Three Rivers Press, 1994.

Kenton, Leslie. *Passage to Power: Natural Menopause Revolution.* Carlsbad, CA: Hay House, 1995.

Lark, Susan M. *Making the Estrogen Decision: All the Information You Need to Make It—Including the Full Range of Natural Alternatives.* New Canaan, CT: Keats Publishing, 1996.

———. *The Menopause Self-Help Book: A Woman's Guide to Feeling Wonderful for the Second Half of Her Life.* Berkeley, CA: Celestial Arts, 1990.

Laucella, Linda. *Hormone Replacement Therapy: Conventional Medicine and Natural Alternatives—Your Guide to Menopausal Health Care Choices.* Los Angeles: Lowell House, 1994.

Laux, Marcus, and Christine Conrad. *Natural Woman, Natural Menopause.* New York: Harper Perennial, 1997.

Love, Susan M., and Karen Lindsey. *Dr. Susan Love's Hormone Book: Making Informed Choices About Menopause.* New York: Times Books, 1997.

Maas, Paula, Susan Brown, and Nancy Bruning. *Natural Medicine for Menopause and Beyond.* New York: Lynn Sonberg/Dell Publishing, 1997.

Mayo, Mary Ann, and Joseph L. Mayo. *The Menopause Manager: A Safe Path for a Natural Change.* Grand Rapids, MI: Fleming H. Revell, 1998.

Murray, Michael T. *Menopause: How You Can Benefit from Diet, Vi-*

tamins, Minerals, Herbs, Exercise, and Other Natural Methods.
Rocklin, CA: Prima Publishing, 1994.

Perry, Susan, and Kate O'Hanlan. *Natural Menopause: The Complete Guide.* Reading, MA: Perseus Books, 1997.

Rinzler, Carol Ann. *Estrogen and Breast Cancer: A Warning to Women.* New York: Macmillan, 1993.

Ryneveld, Edna Copeland. *Secrets of a Natural Menopause: A Positive Drug-Free Approach.* St. Paul, MN: Llewellyn Press, 1994.

Sheehy, Gail. *The Silent Passage.* New York: Random House, 1991.

Stolar, Dr. Mark. *Estrogen: Answers to All Your Questions About Hormone Replacement Therapy and Natural Alternatives.* New York: Avon Books, 1997.

Stoppard, Miriam. *Natural Menopause.* New York: DK Publishing, 1998.

Wilson, Robert. *Feminine Forever.* New York: M. Evans, 1966.

Wright, Jonathan V., and John Morgenthaler. *Natural Hormone Replacement: For Women over Forty-five.* Petaluma, CA: Smart Publications, 1997.

SELECTED ARTICLES FROM GENERAL PERIODICALS AND MEDICAL JOURNALS

Antunes, Carlos. "Endometrial Cancer and Estrogen Use." *New England Journal of Medicine* 300, no. 1 (January 4, 1979), pp. 9–13.

Begley, Sharon, "Understanding Perimenopause"; Marc Peyser, "The Estrogen Dilemma" and "Another Road to Good Health"; Stephen Williams, "You Can Prevent Osteoporosis"; and Karen Springen, "Making Calories Count." *Newsweek* Special Issue, Health for Life, Spring–Summer 1999.

Bergkvist, Leif. "The Risk of Breast Cancer After Estrogen and Estrogen-Progestin Replacement." *New England Journal of Medicine* 321, no. 5 (August 3, 1989), pp. 293–97.

"Bone-Bolstering Combination." *Consumer Reports on Health* 5, no. 5 (May 1993), p. 52.

"Breast Cancer and Long-Term Estrogen Therapy." *Ob/Gyn Clinical Alert* 12, no. 10 (February 1996), pp. 73–80.

Brinton, Louise, Robert Hoover, Moyses Szklo, and Joseph Fraumeni, Jr. "Menopausal Estrogen Use and Risk of Breast Cancer." *Cancer* 47 (1981), pp. 2517–22.

Brody, Jane. "On Menopause and the Toll That Loss of Estrogens Can Take on a Woman's Sexuality." *The New York Times,* May 10, 1990, p. B7.

Chenoy, R. "Effect of Oral Gamolenic Acid from Evening Primrose Oil on Menopausal Flushing." *British Medical Journal* 308, no. 6927 (February 19, 1994).

Chrebet, Jennifer. "More Ways to Keep Bones Strong." *American Health* 14, no. 5 (June 1995), p. 92.

"Coffee Drinkers Require More Dietary Calcium." *Better Nutrition for Today's Living* 56, no. 5 (May 1994), p. 22.

Colditz, Graham. "Hormone Replacement Therapy and Risk of Breast Cancer: Results of Epidemiologic Studies." *American Journal of Obstetrics and Gynecology* 168, no. 5 (May 1993), p. 1473.

Dupont, William. "Estrogen Replacement Therapy and Risk of Breast Cancer" (Editorial Letters). *Journal of the American Medical Association* 265, no. 14 (April 10, 1991), p. 1824.

"The Estrogen Question." *Consumer Reports,* September 1991, pp. 587–91.

Ettinger, B. "Gynecologic Consequences of Long-Term Unopposed Estrogen Replacement Therapy." *Maturitas* 10 (1988), p. 271.

"Exercise Increases Bone Mineral Content of Spine." *National Institute on Aging Special Report on Aging* (1987).

Harting, G. H., C. Moore, and R. Mitchell. "Relationship of Menopausal Status and Exercise Level to HDL Cholesterol in Women." *Experimental Aging Research* 10, no. 1 (1984), pp. 13–18.

Henderson, Brian. "The Cancer Question: An Overview of Recent Epidemiologic and Retrospective Data." *American Journal of Obstetrics and Gynecology* 161, no. 6 (December 1989), pp. 1859–64.

Henderson, Nancy. "Saving Your Skin." *Changing Times,* July 1988, pp. 59–63.

MacPherson, Kathleen. "Menopause as Disease: The Social Construction of a Metaphor." *Advances in Nursing Science* 3, no. 2 (January 1981), pp. 95–113.

Matthews, Karen. "Influences of Natural Menopause on Psychological Characteristics and Symptoms of Middle-Aged Healthy Women." *Journal of Consulting and Clinical Psychology* 58, no. 3 (1990), pp. 345–51.

Neugarten, Bernice L., and Ruth Kraines. "Menopause Symptoms in Women of Various Ages." *Psychosomatic Medicine* 27 (1965), pp. 266–73.

Ross, Ronald, and Annlia Paganini-Hill. "A Case Control Study of Menopausal Estrogen Therapy and Breast Cancer." *Journal of the American Medical Association* 243, no. 16 (April 25, 1980), pp. 1635–39.

Seachrist, Lisa. "What Risk Hormones? Conflicting Studies Reveal Problems in Pinning Down Breast Cancer Risks." *Science News* 148, no. 6 (August 5, 1995), p. 94.

"Some Calcium Supplements Are Found to Be Ineffective." *The New York Times,* March 27, 1987, p. 114.

Whitten, Phillips, and Elizabeth Whiteside. "Can Exercise Make You Sexier?" *Psychology Today,* April 1989, pp. 42–44.

Worcester, Nancy, and Marianne H. Whatley. "The Selling of HRT: Playing on the Fear Factor." *Feminist Review* 41 (Summer 1992), pp. 1–26.

INTERNET RESEARCH AND SUPPORT SITES

There are literally thousands of Internet sites and home pages that either are dedicated to menopause or include information about it. If you type in "menopause" at any of the popular search engines, you will have sites to visit for weeks. Here are a handful of my favorites to get you going.

iVillage.com
An encyclopedic women's site that has more than three hundred articles about menopause. *www.ivillage.com*

Menopause and Beyond
A forum for women who believe that menopause is a normal transition in life. *www.oxford.net/-tishy/beyond.html*

Menopause Support Group
One of the largest discussion and support sites. *members.aol.com/MenoChat/*

National Institutes of Health
Answers to many common questions and a well-balanced discussion on hormones. *www.nih.gov/health/chip/nia/menop/men1.htm*

North American Menopause Society
The comprehensive general resource site of a leading nonprofit scientific organization. *www.menopause.org/*

OnHealth.com

A general medical and health site, with some good articles on menopause, including "Menopausal Problems" *(www.on-health.com/ch1/resource/conditions/item,413.asp)* and "Estrogen—Pros and Cons" *(www.onhealth.com/ch1/in-depth/item/item,1945_1_1.asp). www.onhealth.com*

Power Surge

An online network for women in menopause. *www.power-surge.com/intro.htm*

TRISHA POSNER was involved in fashion and music for twenty years and, at different times, managed boutiques in London and New York, created her own menswear collection, ran the art department for a recording label, and modeled. For the past ten years, she has been researcher and webmaster for her husband, Gerald, on seven books. This is her first solo effort. She lives in New York City. More information is available at www.posner.com.